Losing the
LAST 5 KG

D1350115

To Mum and Dad,

Whose constant self sacrifice and unconditional
love and support allow me the energy, time and
space needed to continue to reach my goals.

To you I dedicate this work.

Losing the
LAST 5 KG

Simple steps
TO GET THE BODY
YOU WANT NOW

Susie Burrell

hardie grant books

Contents

GETTING STARTED

Find your focus **10**

Shift your mindset **12**

Why small changes work **14**

The power of planning **15**

Clean out the cupboards **20**

How to reset your diet the right way **22**

YOUR FOOD

Know your food

Eat more vegetables **30**

Are you eating too many carbs? **36**

The power of protein **44**

Check your good fats **46**

The importance of PUFAs **50**

Avoid the diet food **53**

'Tis sugar, 'tis sugar, 'tis sugar **55**

Liquids

What are you drinking? **60**

Count the coffees **64**

Go 1 month alcohol-free **68**

Snacks

To snack or not to snack? **70**

Nuts once a day **74**

Never leave the house without two vegetables **77**

Know the best treats **78**

Meals

Breakfast success **81**

Get your lunch balance right **88**

The best healthy lunch choices on the go **91**

Halve your dinner **96**

The best low-calorie dinners **97**

Know your quick and easy meals **100**

Soup it up **105**

Learn to love salads **107**

Tricks to make it easier

Embrace a sugar detox **112**

Are you having any extras? **115**

Go smaller **117**

Quality over quantity **121**

Get your timing right **124**

Are the people in your life making you fat? **127**

Be smart when eating out **132**

Take a meal off **138**

YOUR BEHAVIOUR

Check yourself

How many times a day does food enter your mouth? **142**

Know your eating style **143**

Food habits that make you fat **147**

Are your hormones making you fat? **151**

Sustainable change

Reset your hunger switch **154**

Consider a fast **157**

Mindless munching **160**

Develop your self-regulation skills **163**

Build your willpower **165**

Managing cravings **169**

Learn to stop overeating **171**

Think thin **174**

Expect a plateau **178**

YOUR BODY

Start small **182**

Measure your body **184**

Get a pedometer **186**

Start training **188**

Learn to interval train **190**

Time to lift **191**

Check your calories **193**
Fuel your body for training **198**
Is working out making you fatter? **201**

YOUR LIFE

Work

Take control of your office food habits **206**
Manage your stress **209**
Travel smart **213**

Home

Get a daily timetable **215**
Sacred Sunday **217**

Moving forward

You have the power to manage your weight **218**
Victim no more **219**
No more excuses **221**
Rejecting laziness **226**
See only solutions **227**
Commit to self-care **229**
Commit to a steely mindset **230**
Cement your new habits **232**
Maintain your motivation **235**
Embrace your true self **237**

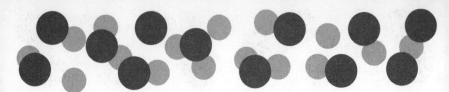

getting STARTED

'You've wasted enough time and energy on diets that get you nowhere. The time to get your food, your behaviour, your body and your life under control is now.'

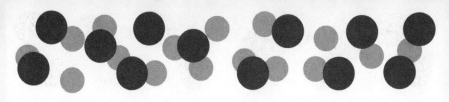

Find your focus   10

Shift your mindset   12

Why small changes work   14

The power of planning   15

Clean out the cupboards   20

How to reset your diet the
   right way   22

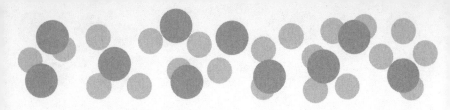

Find your focus

'You are either committed to losing weight or you are not. There is nothing in between.'

One of the main reasons that many of us carry around extra weight is that it's so easy to gradually put on. It's easy to ignore, relatively easy to cover up and very easy to tell ourselves that such a small amount of extra weight doesn't really matter. We will lose it eventually.

To some extent we may be kidding ourselves, but when push comes to shove, if we set our minds to it, it's actually quite easy to lose the extra weight if we find and maintain our focus for a decent amount of time. Of course it would be nice to drop it in a few days, but when weight is lost that quickly it's generally water – not fat – and rarely achieved via sustainable methods. But if you're happy to spend just a few weeks minus your worst food habits and high-calorie treats, it's possible to lose – and keep off – your extra weight.

This book has been designed as both a quick-tip guide to dip into for those who already have a reasonably healthy lifestyle and just need a few tricks to get back on track, or as a full program from start to finish for those who need to go right back to the drawing board. In my experience working with weight-loss clients for almost 20 years, it's not the super strict regimes that achieve sustainable weight loss long-term. It's the small but significant

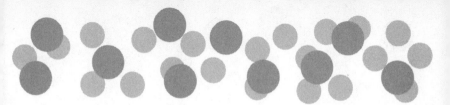

changes we can maintain for life that see weight gradually shift for good. No matter what your starting point is as you grab this book, you will find useful tips and tricks that help you lose the weight for good.

Before you use this book as yet another weight loss program that you follow for a few days before becoming bored and reverting to your midmorning banana bread and caramel latte habit, can you commit the next 2–4 weeks to making a serious dent in your extra weight? Are you ready to prioritise your training so you don't skip your gym session, again? Are you ready to avoid your diet-saboteur friends who offer you chocolates at work? Are you ready to rid yourself of your life-long diet mindset, which has taught you to believe that you have a slow metabolism and that you cannot lose weight? Are you ready to feel good?

While weight loss does not require you to be a diet and exercise purist, during the initial stages the more strict you are the better the immediate results will be. A small but significant weight loss experienced in the first few weeks of a new dietary regime is all you need to stay motivated and on track.

So, to move forward, clear your diary and get ready to commit to a good few weeks of healthy eating, exercise and taking control of your extra weight, once and for all.

Shift your mindset

'You have got to make conscious choices every day to shed the old – old issues, old guilt and old patterns.'

While most of us know how to eat well and stay healthy, it's often easier said than done. Busy lifestyles and family demands regularly result in health and fitness pursuits being put on the back burner, but it's our small, daily food and exercise choices that determine successful weight control. Fad diets, weight-loss challenges and boot camps may all have some short-term benefits for the mind and the body, but until health and fitness is viewed as a way of life as opposed to a short-term commitment, you are likely to find yourself back to where you started – signing up for yet another diet craze that takes you nowhere.

Once you prioritise looking after your body as part of your daily routine, the decisions that impact on your health are a whole lot easier to make. You don't even have to think about them. Instead of buying a pile of expensive, unappealing diet food on impulse to support a new fad regime, you automatically set aside time each week to buy the food your body needs to be at its best. You no longer have to deprive yourself of sweet treats because your desire to eat them has reduced. And most importantly, when you have indulged for a special occasion, you know what you need to do in order to get yourself back on track quickly.

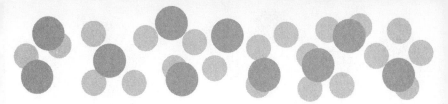

Achieving the motivation and focus to implement such lifestyle changes develops gradually. First you need to admit that you are not feeling 100 per cent, and decide that you would look and feel much better if taking care of your body was part of your daily routine. Fuelling it with good-quality food, moving it regularly and keeping your intake of high-fat, highly processed foods to a minimum needs to become a habit, and the motivation to build and cement this habit has to come from somewhere deep within. Only this will drive you to do the things your body needs to be at its best, every single day.

To make changes to your health and fitness mindset, start by observing your current health-related behaviour. Take a look at your body in the mirror and see the evidence of where you have not been taking care of it. Think about how much better you would feel if you were fitter, or had less weight to carry each day. Then consider the easiest and most important changes you can make. Do you need to eat more vegetables and rely less on takeaway food? Are you choosing to drink water or sugar-laden soft drinks? Day to day, each food choice and exercise habit you reinforce contributes to your body shape and fitness level. Motivation does not come from following the latest fad diet, nor does it come from your partner, kids or workmates. It has to come from somewhere deep within and ultimately become the thing that drives you to do the things your body needs to be at its best, every single day.

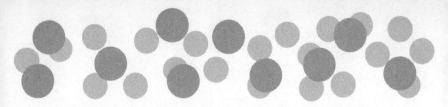

Why small changes work

'It's not the occasional burger or chocolate that ruins your diet – your daily routine controls your weight long-term.'

We have all tried them – ridiculously strict, exhausting diets that we stick to for a few days or even weeks before we eat something taboo and throw it all in. Introducing small dietary changes and regular exercise is a much more achievable alternative. While you will not see dramatic weight loss each week, unlike the various soup and shake programs you have tried before, you will feel better by losing a smaller amount but being able to keep it off.

Too often we overcommit ourselves, becoming slaves to unreasonable goals and feeling disappointed and frustrated when we don't achieve them. We expect to lose weight in an instant, train for hours on top of long working hours and family commitments, have a buzzing social life, and prepare restaurant-style dinners and nutritionally balanced lunches for the following day. No wonder we fail – we set ourselves up for it.

Imagine if you could add one or two positive health changes to your day – snacking on vegetables or keeping your dinner small – and you could feel just as good and be losing weight at the same time. The good news is that you can. While allocating some energy and time to losing weight will help get you started on the right foot, the general rule is to only adopt changes that realistically fit into your life. Sustaining these small changes long-term will add up, and so too will your weight loss.

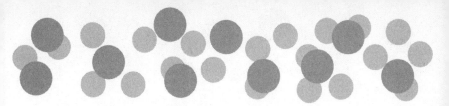

The power of planning

'Planning is the key to dietary success.'

It may surprise you to hear that when it comes to diets, weight control and nutrition, it is planning rather than knowledge that is the key to success. In fact, it is safe to say that most of us know what we should (or should not) be eating – we know that fruit and vegetables are good, and we know that fried food is not so good. We know that chocolate is high in calories, and we know that if we eat less we will lose weight. Knowledge is not the issue.

Rather, in busy, overscheduled lives, our healthy eating regimes fall off track when we find ourselves hungry and without good food choices on hand. Sometimes we may be able to ignore the hunger pains and wait until we stumble across an apple, but in more cases than not the deep desire for food sees us searching desk drawers, attacking vending machines or at the local shop stocking up on high-fat, high-sugar, carbohydrate-rich foods that feed our low blood sugar levels like a drug feeds an addict.

The simple act of planning ensures that we are never caught off guard and always have healthy options on hand to make it easy to eat well. And while some people may opt to spend hours each Sunday packing portion-controlled lunches, the good news is that it does not have to be this labour intensive to get good results.

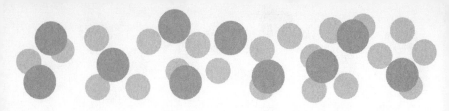

1. SCHEDULE TIME

Often, the greatest barrier to taking control of our food and calorie intake is finding ourselves in a cycle of not having enough time and bouncing from week to week eating whatever crosses our path. The solution to this is easy – all we need to do is schedule time to get organised. All you need is 20–30 minutes each week to plan a few meals, write a shopping list and consider the way your upcoming week will impact your food choices. For example, if you know that you will be home late a couple of nights, you know that you will need a couple of fast, easy meal options that can be heated quickly to avoid you resorting to high-fat takeaway.

2. SHOP ONLINE

If you visit the supermarket several times each week, chances are you are not only purchasing extra foods you do not need, but also wasting plenty of valuable time – parking, queuing and waiting. Shopping online not only saves much time and energy but helps you to plan your meals in advance. There is also the option of ordering a fruit and vegetable box each week to ensure you have fresh staples on hand, or have an array of healthy lunch and snack options delivered straight to your workplace.

3. COOK SMART

In an ideal world we would grow fresh produce in our garden, shop locally and prepare healthy home cooked meals each night. Unfortunately, busy lives are not always conducive to this grassroots approach to our food intake, and fewer and fewer people are finding

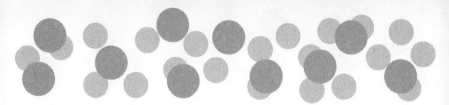

time to cook a healthy meal each night. For this reason, looking at time-efficient ways to prepare meals is the key to success. Try bulk preparing meals in advance so you cook just once or twice each week. This will also free up time on other evenings when you know you will struggle to find the time to cook a meal from scratch.

4. CREATE HABITS

Eating well long-term is about building solid food habits that become your natural default. For example, taking your lunch with you each day, or always keeping a water bottle or healthy snack with you. It takes between 30–90 days to cement a long-term habit, which is why focusing on your nutrition for a set period of time will help to initially identify and solidify the health habits you know you need to build and maintain long-term. Phone or computer reminders and alarms, post-it notes and regular time-outs are all tools that can help you refocus on your daily dietary goals.

5. HAVE BACK-UPS

In life, things rarely go to plan – the time you had set aside for meal preparation gets eaten away by other commitments; your shopping order does not arrive; or, you forget to take your lunch. To help buffer for these regular occurrences when it comes to your nutrition, always have a back-up plan. Keep a healthy frozen meal on hand; know what you can order from the food court if you need; and keep a protein or meal bar in your work bag for emergencies. Remember, your nutrition does not have to be perfect to get good results, it just has to be consistent.

Power planning checklist

1   Shop once a week – if the food is not in the house, you cannot eat it. Set aside an hour each week to stock up on your dietary staples or try ordering online if you find it hard to make it to the shops.

2   Know your quick and easy meals – if you have tuna or salmon, eggs, cheese, pasta sauce, frozen vegetables, potatoes and tomatoes you can make five or six different meals in 10 minutes or less.

3   Cook just once or twice a week – if you prepare a couple of big serves of a nutritionally balanced meal such as a pasta bake, a pie or a stir-fry with meat and vegetables, you are guaranteed two meals during the week and leftovers for your lunch.

4   Start a lunch club – if you are tired of the same old boring sandwich or salad that you bring from home, team up with a work colleague and start a lunch-buddy system. This way you can bring two tasty lunches each week and perhaps shout yourself to lunch out on the fifth day of the week.

5   Set aside 20 minutes on Sunday night to plan meals – make a note of each dish you plan to prepare so you know exactly what you need to do to prepare it when you walk in the door.

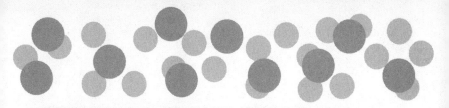

6   Keep snacks with you at all times – each morning pack a couple of protein-rich snack foods to prevent impulse food purchases during the day.

7   Utilise lunchtimes – if you find it difficult to plan your food over the weekend, utilise lunch breaks at work to get to the local supermarket and stock up on the foods you need during the day, and even for the evening meal.

8   Have a cook up – if the weekdays are simply too frantic to prepare any meals, cook a couple of extra meals over the weekend so you are certain to eat well for at least the first few nights of the week.

9   Develop food rules – create clear limits on when you will and will not eat certain types of food. For example, resolve only to eat out twice each week, this way you know when and in what context you will indulge, which will help with your diet goals.

10 Utilise helpers – there are many mums, husbands and friends who are often only too happy to help at home if you need them to. Next time, when one of your support team asks if you need help, ask if they will help you with a meal or leftovers. You will be surprised how happy they will be to help.

Clean out the cupboards

'If you really don't want to eat it, throw it away.'

There are very few people who can keep highly appealing foods such as chocolate biscuits, potato chips and other sweet treats at home without eating them. It's human nature to eat food when we see it. On top of the powerful visual stimulus food provides, we have the many years of food programming, courtesy of our parents, that teaches us from an early age about good and bad foods, and that we should limit the bad ones. This message of restriction quickly translates into wanting what we can't have and the inability to stop eating high-fat, treat foods when they are readily available to us.

A question I often ask my clients is, 'If I came and looked inside your cupboard, would I throw anything out?' In most cases, the answer is yes. The extra biscuits that are kept in case friends visit, the chips that are for parties, the soft drink for the kids. These are foods few of us should be eating but we actively choose to keep them in our visual field as a constant source of temptation.

Clearing out the fridge and the cupboards when you are about to commit to a new lifestyle regime is like a spring clean of your wardrobe. You cannot believe you kept those old daggy clothes around for so long and feel so much better once they're gone. The biscuits, chocolate bars, chips,

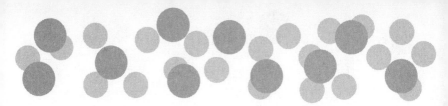

juice and soft drink all have to go. And before you say, 'But they're for the kids,' remember they are not good for the kids either. Once the cleanout is complete, replace the discarded items with key items you need on hand for those late nights returning home. Tuna, eggs, pasta sauce, pasta, low-fat cheese, frozen vegetables and potatoes can be converted into numerous quick, nutritious dinners in just 5–10 minutes.

Actively creating your own healthy environment, whether it's at home, your partner's place or at work, is absolutely crucial if you want to give yourself the best chance of staying on track with your new food regime. Remember, if tempting food is in front of you, you will want to eat it – you are not weak or a glutton, you are simply human. Limiting your exposure to tempting treats is imperative as you strive to reach your diet and lifestyle goals.

DIET CORRUPTORS	CALORIES	CARBS (g)	FAT (g)
250 g block milk chocolate	1300	155	70
100 g cheese	360	0	32
50 g potato chips	260	24	16
1 chocolate biscuit	100	12	5
200 ml fruit juice	80	18	0
10 plain rice crackers	70	15	2

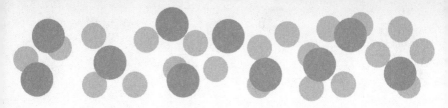

How to reset your diet the right way

'The benefit of a diet reset is that it reminds you how good you feel when you eat well.'

While we regularly hear about diet 'detoxes' and a growing range of fasts, cleanses, juices and detox programs, it is important that we do not get too caught up in the hype – few, if any, of the claims made by such programs are proven, realistic or even true.

The human body does not need to be 'detoxed' – the kidneys, liver and immune system generally do a very good job of getting rid of the nasties on a daily basis. There is not one product or nutrient that holds the answer to any health issue that may develop. The human body is made up of a complex, intricate system of cellular metabolic functions and processes that we are unlikely to ever understand completely.

In saying that, what we do know about weight loss and diets in general is that when individuals get immediate results they are more likely to continue with a new regime, and a relatively strict period of healthy eating can result in a quick drop on the scales. For this reason, adopting a brief period of time in which natural, whole foods are consumed with the goal of 'cleaning out' your diet and dropping a few kilos is not a bad thing. In

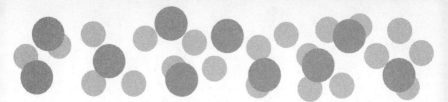

fact, anything that reminds you how much better you feel when you are eating well can only be considered a good outcome. The key is to know how to kickstart your diet the right way.

COMMIT FOR A BRIEF PERIOD OF TIME

Generally speaking, there is no issue with eating only fresh fruit and vegetables for a short period of time, say three to five days. After this period of time, the nutrients the body requires to function optimally (including protein, iron, zinc and calcium) should be reincorporated into the diet. Extreme diets that encourage fasting or eliminating several food groups for long periods of time are associated with a number of issues including reduced metabolic rate. For this reason, they are not advisable for the vast majority of active, busy people. Committing to a diet detox for a week or less – a time in which you have no social engagements – can keep you 100 per cent focused on your nutrition.

BASE YOUR MEALS AROUND FRESH FRUIT AND VEGETABLES

A diet detox does not need to be complicated, it can simply be a few days of eating only fresh, unprocessed foods. The simple goal of basing all of your meals for this time around fresh fruit and vegetables – soups, salads, stir-fries, smoothies and juices – will seriously load your body full of vitamins, minerals and fibre. It will help to eliminate the body of excess fluid and allow you to drop a kilogram or two without skipping meals or drinking only juice.

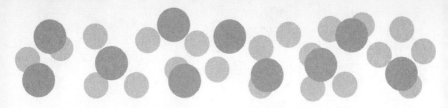

DROP THE SNACKS

Generally speaking, we eat far too much, far too often and rarely feel hungry in between our meals. Shifting our dietary pattern away from eating every couple of hours to leaving 4–5 hours between meals is an easy way to kickstart our metabolism and get into the habit of eating balanced, filling meals 3–4 times each day. Cutting out snacks also automatically eliminates a number of processed, high-carb foods from our daily diets including crackers, muffins, milk coffees, biscuits and snack bars.

DRINK ONLY WATER

Another simple way to reset your diet is to focus on drinking a couple of litres of water each day along with herbal teas in place of your regular caffeine-rich drinks and high-sugar juices and smoothies. Not only is this an easy way to significantly reduce your calorie intake, but focusing on optimal hydration is an easy way to get your digestive system working efficiently. It will also have you looking and feeling at your best each day.

UTILISE SOUP

Generally speaking, any diet that contains fewer calories than you are used to leaves you vulnerable to hunger. A simple trick to avoid this, especially during the initial stages of a detox, is to eat a thick vegetable soup to provide bulk without many calories. A vegetable soup based on leek, celery, onions and garlic will not only provide nutrition but also help to draw excess fluid from the body, leaving you feeling light and less bloated. Try replacing both lunch and dinner with a vegetable soup for a couple of days at the beginning of your detox (see recipe on next page).

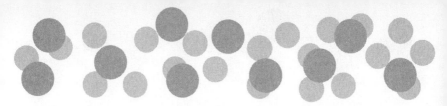

DETOX SOUP

2 teaspoons olive oil

1 onion, finely chopped

1 leek, white part only, washed and finely sliced

½ head of celery, chopped

2 cups (500 ml) salt-reduced vegetable stock

3 cups (750 ml) water

400 g tin chopped tomatoes

1 carrot, cut into 1 cm cubes

500 g pumpkin, peeled and cut into 1 cm cubes

1 head of broccoli, cut into florets and steamed

1 Gently heat the oil in a large saucepan. Add the onion, leek and celery and sauté over a low heat for about 5 minutes, or until soft.

2 Add the stock, water, tomatoes, carrot and pumpkin. Bring to the boil, then reduce the heat and simmer for 10 minutes.

3 Top with the steamed broccoli and serve.

Serves 6–8

Top 10 tips for a successful detox

1   Eliminate all alcohol and caffeine, including tea, coffee and cola drinks.

2   Eliminate all processed snack foods, such as biscuits, bars, cakes and cereals.

3   Eat at least 3 cups of vegetables or salad and 2 pieces of fruit each day.

4   Snack on fresh fruit or a handful of nuts.

5   Stick to lean proteins, such as chicken breast with vegetables/salad for main meals.

6   Include at least 1 cup of wholegrain carbohydrates each day for energy. Good choices include oats, beans, chickpeas and sweet potato.

7   Expect to feel tired and headachy for the first couple of days before feeling revitalised by day three.

8   Aim to drink 2–3 litres of water each day. More than this is not necessarily better.

9   Don't over-train during your detox – a 30–60 minute walk each day is more than adequate when you are not eating many calories.

10 Commit to a detox period of just 5–7 days.

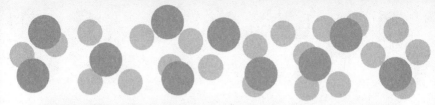

SAMPLE WEEKLY DETOX PLAN

	MONDAY	TUESDAY	WEDNESDAY	THURSDAY	FRIDAY
BREAKFAST	Vegetable juice + large bowl fruit salad	Vegetable juice + 200 g natural yoghurt + fresh berries + sprinkle of walnuts	Vegetable juice + ⅓ cup oats + 1 cup low-fat milk	Vegetable juice + ⅓ cup oats + 1 cup low-fat milk	Vegetarian omelette
MID MORNING	Piece of fruit	Piece of fruit	Piece of fruit	Piece of fruit	Piece of fruit
LUNCH	Detox soup	Detox soup	½ cup brown rice + small tin tuna + sweet chilli sauce	Detox soup	Chicken salad
MID AFTERNOON	Handful of almonds + 1 piece of fresh fruit	Handful of almonds + 1 piece of fresh fruit	2 corn thins + 2 teaspoons no added sugar peanut butter	30 g mixed nuts + 1 piece of fruit	2 corn thins + 2 teaspoons no added sugar peanut butter
DINNER	Detox soup	150 g white fish + detox soup	150 g grilled fish or chicken breast + mixed vegetables	Prawn and vegetable stir-fry with ½ cup brown rice	Detox soup

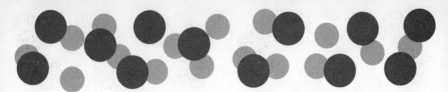

your FOOD

'Your body is a temple that deserves to be
nourished with good food.'

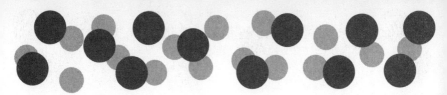

KNOW YOUR FOOD

Eat more vegetables	30
Are you eating too many carbs?	36
The power of protein	44
Check your good fats	46
The importance of PUFAs	50
Avoid the diet food	53
'Tis sugar, 'tis sugar, 'tis sugar	55

LIQUIDS

What are you drinking?	60
Count the coffees	64
Go 1 month alcohol-free	68

SNACKS

To snack or not to snack?	70
Nuts once a day	74
Never leave the house without two vegetables	77
Know the best treats	78

MEALS

Breakfast success	81
Get your lunch balance right	88
The best healthy lunch choices on the go	91
Halve your dinner	96
The best low-calorie dinners	97
Know your quick and easy meals	100
Soup it up	105
Learn to love salads	107

TRICKS TO MAKE IT EASIER

Embrace a sugar detox	112
Are you having any extras?	115
Go smaller	117
Quality over quantity	121
Get your timing right	124
Are the people in your life making you fat?	127
Be smart when eating out	132
Take a meal off	138

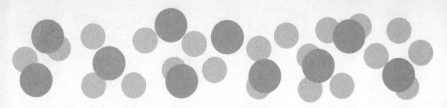

Eat more vegetables

'Just one piece of advice for better health and weight control – eat more vegetables.'

Of all the scientific evidence that points to keeping healthy and our body weight in check, eating plenty of vegetables wins hands down. It is also safe to say that the majority of us know that vegetables are good for us, so why do we not eat more of them?

When things get busy, for a number of reasons, it is the vegetable component of our evening meal that falls by the wayside. Meals purchased on the run or that are prepared quickly at home are often light on fresh vegetables – the downside of which is that we fail to get all the fibre, vitamins, minerals and bulk in the diet that we need to feel full and satisfied, leaving us prone to overeating.

Ideally an adult requires at least 3 cups of vegetables or salad every day, and the brighter the colour of the vegetables, the better they will be for you. Unlike fruit, which is carbohydrate-based, most vegetables consist mainly of water so have virtually no calories, which means you can eat as many as you like without fear of weight gain. Eating plenty of nutrient-rich vegetables daily also means that you simply have less room in your diet for poor-quality food.

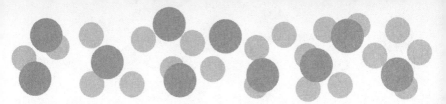

Diets rich in brightly coloured, fresh vegetables also have enormous benefits for cell health. Vegetables contain a complex array of phytochemicals, antioxidants and minerals that work in unison to protect cells from the damage linked to ageing, macular degeneration and even some types of cancer. While there are literally hundreds of supplementary forms of these nutrients, the evidence to date suggests that the health benefits are strongest when the real food forms are eaten.

In order to get enough vegetables in your daily diet, you need to have serves at both lunch and dinner. Order or make your sandwiches with lots of salad, or take an extra couple of salad vegetables with you to eat with your lunch. Juicing vegetables including carrots, celery and beetroot is another great way to incorporate them into your diet. Try enjoying them in soup for a lunch option or even raw as a pre-dinner snack. Dinner plates should be routinely half-filled with vegetables or salad. Make a concerted effort to always order extra sides of vegetables or salad when eating out.

By simply focusing on increasing the vegetable content of your daily diet, you can reduce your total caloric intake without even noticing.

Top 10 ways to eat more vegetables

1   **Order them online** One of the biggest barriers to eating
    enough fresh produce is having it readily available at home. If you
    regularly find yourself running out, perhaps it is worth considering
    a weekly online order from your local market. Not only is this
    a cost-effective solution, you are guaranteed seasonal, fresh
    produce delivered to your door.

2   **Have back ups** Frozen or tinned vegetables are a great back up
    and can be just as good nutritionally as fresh vegetables if cooked
    correctly. Steam frozen vegetables lightly and use minimal water,
    as the vitamins will leach into the water as they are being cooked.
    Frozen peas, carrots and broccoli can be added to most dishes.

3   **Cut them up immediately** If you cut up vegetables and place
    them in a bowl in the fridge or middle of the kitchen bench, you
    will find the whole family munches on them just because they
    are there.

4   **Half-the-plate rule** Remember, half your dinner plate should
    be filled with salad or vegetables – no exceptions.

5   **Add them at lunch** Plain wraps, sandwiches, crackers and
    sushi are healthy lunch choices but they will not be supplying
    the amount of bulk from vegetables and salad that you need. Try
    adding an extra tomato, some cucumber or capsicum to your
    lunch and notice how much more satisfied you feel.

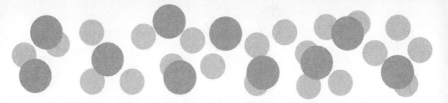

6 **Order extra when eating out** Most restaurants and takeaway options will not include enough vegetables. Always order extra sides of vegetables to balance your meal nutritionally.

7 **The 5 pm munchies** Many of us overindulge in dips, potato chips and other tasty nibbles at the end of the day, especially as we are preparing dinner. When the late afternoon munchies hit, try snacking on crunchy fresh vegetables with low-fat dip. Not only will you fill yourself up so you don't overeat at dinner, you will have taken care of a couple of serves of vegetables for that day.

8 **Dress them up** Vegetables don't have to be served steamed or soggy with no flavour. There is nothing wrong with baking them in a little olive oil, serving with a light cheese sauce or stir-frying with a small amount of oyster or hoisin sauce for flavour – don't be scared of making them taste good.

9 **Soup or salad?** Studies have shown that starting the meal with a vegetable broth or salad can reduce your calorie intake at the main meal by up to 20 per cent!

10 **Juice it** If all else fails, a vegetable juice made with no fruit is an extremely nutritious addition to the day – so start juicing!

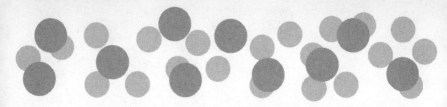

VEGETABLE STACKS

1 butternut pumpkin, peeled and
cut into chunks

2 zucchini

2 tablespoons olive oil

1 large eggplant

1 red capsicum

4 large field mushrooms,
stems removed

1 garlic clove, finely chopped

200 g asparagus, lightly blanched

100 g low-fat fetta cheese

Serves 4

1 Preheat the oven to 180°C. Microwave the pumpkin until soft enough to slice, for about 3–5 minutes. Slice the pumpkin and zucchini into thin strips lengthways, brush with some of the oil and place on a baking tray. Bake for 10–20 minutes, or until tender.

2 Cut the eggplant into rounds and capsicum into quarters. Brush with the remaining oil and place on a baking tray. Bake for 5–10 minutes, or until tender.

3 Assemble the baked vegetables into 4 stacks on a baking tray. Sit a mushroom on top of each stack. Sprinkle the garlic over the mushroom.

4 Place the stacks back in the oven and bake for about 5–10 minutes, until the mushroom is warmed through.

5 Serve with asparagus spears and crumbled fetta.

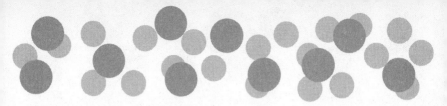

CHEESY VEGETABLE BAKE

500 g cauliflower, cut into small florets

500 g broccoli, cut into small florets

1 onion, finely chopped

1 garlic clove, finely chopped

2 slices of low-fat bacon, chopped

1 teaspoon olive oil

¼ cup plain flour

2½ cups (625 ml) low-fat milk

¾ cup grated low-fat cheddar cheese

Serves 4–6

1 Preheat the oven to 180°C. Lightly steam the cauliflower and broccoli until just tender. Place in a baking dish.

2 In a saucepan, sauté the onion, garlic and bacon in oil over a medium heat until the onion is soft.

3 Add the flour and cook, stirring, over a low heat for about 1 minute, until smooth. Slowly stir in the milk and bring to the boil, then simmer uncovered for 5–10 minutes, stirring until the sauce is thick. Stir in the cheese.

4 Pour the sauce over the vegetables in the baking dish. Bake for 15–20 minutes, or until heated through.

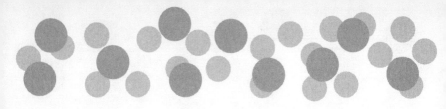

Are you eating too many carbs?

'Carbs are not bad for us, it is simply about the type, how much we need and how much we are actually having.'

If there was just one dietary area in which the thinking has changed significantly in recent years it would have to be the area of carbohydrates. Long gone are the days of a low-fat, high-carb diet; nowadays carbs are often avoided. So, are carbs really that bad for you, how much is too much, and which carbs should you be eating?

Carbohydrates are primarily found in plant-based foods including bread, rice, breakfast cereal, fruit, starchy vegetables and sugars. They contain 4 calories of energy per gram. The simplest form of carbohydrate is glucose. Carbohydrates range from mixes of simple sugars to hundreds of individual sugars which form more complex carbohydrates, such as breads and cereals. Carbohydrates can also be grouped according to their glycaemic index. The glycaemic index refers to how quickly a carbohydrate releases glucose into the bloodstream. Carbohydrate-based foods that release glucose more slowly into the blood stream – such as legumes, wholegrain bread and stone fruit – are low GI foods. High GI foods – such as white bread, rice and tropical fruit – release the glucose they contain relatively quickly into the blood stream.

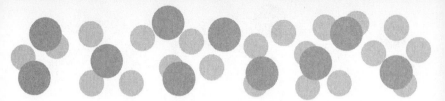

Generally speaking, natural sources of carbohydrate as found in fruit, starchy vegetables, legumes and wholegrains are the best sources of carbohydrate in the diet. Here they are consumed as part of whole foods, offer a range of other key nutrients including fibre, vitamins and minerals, and are far less likely to be overconsumed the way refined carbohydrates (including processed cereals, white breads and biscuits) are.

Traditionally it was recommended that active individuals primarily base their intake around carbohydrate-rich foods simply because carbohydrates are the primary fuel for the muscle. As such, the more active an individual, the greater the amount of carbohydrate they will require to adequately fuel their muscles. Modern thinking has changed in this view slightly: while individuals may be relatively active for some parts of the day, many of us also spend many hours sitting, which means our carbohydrate requirements are significantly reduced.

ISN'T LOW-CARB BETTER FOR FAT LOSS?

As carbs are the primary fuel for the muscles, it is a common belief that eating fewer carbs means that you automatically burn a greater amount of fat. While this is somewhat true (the body prefers to burn carbs in the form of glucose as its primary energy source), if carbs are restricted to a significant extent your body will shift to burning fat but will also slow metabolic rate over time. This means that initially you will get good results from a strict low-carb approach but over time, as your metabolic rate reduces, the body will be burning fewer calories overall. This effect

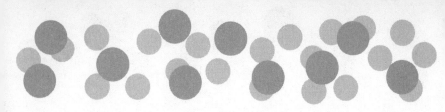

can be observed in individuals who have great success initially using a low-carb approach but who find it difficult to maintain or achieve again once they return to their usual carbohydrate intake.

HOW MUCH CARBOHYDRATE DO I NEED?

The amount of carbs we need largely depends on how much we move: if you spend all day on your feet and are already quite slim, you will need more than someone who sits all day, does not work out and who has insulin resistance. Similarly, on days you train for an hour or more, you will need more than on a sedentary day when you barely leave the house. A high-carb diet is useful for those training more than two hours a day, such as young athletes. A low-carb diet is useful for those who lead more sedentary lifestyles, training less than one hour a day, or those who want to lose weight. As a general rule, someone training an hour a day will lose ½–1 kg a week with 30–40 per cent of calories coming from carbs, which equates to 20–30 g carbs at both breakfast and lunch, followed by a taper towards the second half of the day.

Now while this is all good in theory, when it comes to actual eating behaviours, people understand these approaches very differently. They may think they are eating 'low-carb', but they are often eating the wrong balance of carbs throughout the day. Perhaps they are not eating enough at breakfast and then overdoing things with heavy rice or quinoa salads at lunch, or extra snacks, coffees and juices throughout the day. The timing and proportion of the carbs you eat are just as important as the total amount.

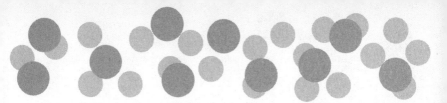

When it comes to weight control, it is important to know that the amount of carbohydrate in different types of food differs widely. For example, a couple of slices of bread can contain as little as 20 g of total carbs per two slices and up to as much as 80 g of carbs – depending on the slice size, thickness and density. For this reason, becoming more aware of how much total carbohydrate you are consuming helps to inform ways in which it can be dramatically reduced in order to support weight loss.

One of the easiest ways to understand your own carbohydrate intake is to work out how much you are consuming via a dietary app that counts the grams of carbohydrates you are consuming. An average, active female will lose weight consuming 100–140 g of total carbs per day, while a male (who will require a little more), can lose weight consuming 140–180 g per day. Any less tends to see halted weight loss results as the total amount of fuel is a little too low.

Once you gain some insight into how much carbohydrate you are consuming on average each day, you can adjust the amounts depending on your weight loss goals. For example, if you are consuming just 100 g of total carbohydrate each day, you may need an extra 20–40 g, while if you calculate that you are consuming a lot more than this, you can cut back a little.

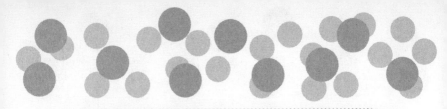

Carb counter

Sample 20 g carb serves:
1 medium jacket potato
½ cup sweet potato
½ corn cob
½ cup cooked rice
½ cup cooked pasta
¾ cup kidney beans/chickpeas
½ cup quinoa
2 slices low-carb bread
1 piece of fruit
1 regular milk coffee
250 ml juice

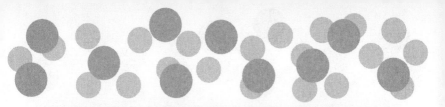

	SAMPLE CARB DIETS	
MEAL	**HIGH-CARB DIET** **~50–60% CARBS,** **20–25% PROTEIN,** **25–30% FAT**	**REDUCED CARB DIET** **30–40% CARBS,** **~30–40% PROTEIN,** **20–30% FAT**
BREAKFAST	Wholegrain cereal with milk and a banana	2 eggs and 1 slice wholegrain toast
SNACK	Fruit yoghurt	Cheese and wholegrain crackers
LUNCH	Bread roll with tuna or tuna pasta	Salad with tuna and ½ cup sweet potato
SNACK	Energy bar/fruit	Handful of nuts and 1 piece of fruit
DINNER	150 g lean meat, 2–3 cups pasta/rice and vegetables	175 g lean meat and 2–3 cups vegetables
DESSERT	Fruit and yoghurt	

Getting your carb balance right

1   **The more grains the better** The more grains your bread,
    cereal or crackers have, the better they will be for you. Grain-based
    products have some of the lowest GI values, so are digested slowly
    and will leave you feeling full for longer.

2   **Measure your serves** The main issue with rice, pasta, noodles
    and breakfast cereal is not the amount of carbohydrate that they
    contain, but how much of them we eat. Aim for just ½–1 cup of
    cooked carbohydrates with your meals.

3   **Go for smaller slices** Have you noticed how much bigger
    slices of bread are getting? Some of the slices are so large they
    don't fit in the toaster. Choose the smallest slices of bread you can
    find and you will be eating up to 20 g of carbohydrate less every
    time you eat 2 slices of bread.

4   **Choose your breakfast cereals carefully** Unfortunately
    there are few breakfast cereals on the market that have a low GI.
    Muesli, oats and bran are among the few, which means that the
    popular flakes, rice cereals, honey and chocolate flavoured
    varieties need to go.

5   **Always eat carbs and protein together** The GI of
    carbohydrate-containing foods is heavily influenced by what
    foods you eat with them. Aiming for lean protein from meat, fish,
    low-fat dairy or beans with your carbohydrate will naturally lower
    the glycaemic response and help keep you fuller for longer. Good
    examples are wholegrain crackers with low-fat cheese, yoghurt
    with fruit, or rice with tuna.

6 **Be careful with '97% fat free'** In many cases, lowering the fat content means that biscuits, crackers, yoghurts and snack foods have had more sugar added to compensate, which increases their GI value. Such processed foods tend to offer little nutritionally and leave you prone to overeating.

7 **Eat more beans** Legumes including baked beans, chickpeas, kidney beans and lentils have some of the lowest GI ratings. Add to minced meat dishes, salads and stir-fries to bulk up the meal with fibre and protein.

8 **Count the times you eat** The body is designed to eat and then wait at least 2–3 hours before eating again. Constant grazing on milk-based coffees, biscuits and fruit can really disrupt the natural digestive processes and make it difficult to lose weight. Stick to your meals and midmeals and stop snacking in between.

9 **If in doubt, go for brown** If you are unsure of the GI of a food, choosing the brown or wholemeal option is generally better. While not all wholemeal products have a low GI, you will still be getting the benefits of extra protein and fibre.

10 **Be smart with fruit** Of course fruit is a healthy food choice at any time of the day but fruit does have a carbohydrate and calorie load, which means you cannot eat as much as you like. Aim for 2–3 pieces of fruit each day as a snack with yoghurt or nuts, or after meals, and remember the brighter the colour of the fruit, the better it will be for you.

The power of protein

'Protein helps you avoid those sugar highs and lows that leave you prone to overeating.'

Protein, thanks to the numerous Hollywood celebrities who swear by their high-protein regimes, has been the diet buzzword of the decade. Protein is thought to have several benefits for weight control as it is nutrient-rich and keeps you full for longer, and hence more likely to stick to your diet.

Protein contains 4 calories of energy per gram, the same as carbohydrate, and is found in largest amounts in animal products, including meat, chicken, fish and dairy, as well as in soy, nuts and whole grains in smaller amounts. Protein is used for muscle repair, to build skin and hair and to provide essential amino acids that are involved in a number of chemical processes in the body. As proteins are not primarily used as a fuel source, they are also digested after carbohydrates and hence thought to play a powerful role in inducing feelings of satiety or fullness.

POWERFUL PROTEIN CHOICES		
MEAL	**TYPICAL CHOICE**	**HIGHER PROTEIN CHOICE**
Breakfast	Toast with jam	Toast with 1 egg
Midmorning	Fruit	Low-fat cheese and crackers
Lunch	Peanut butter sandwich	50 g turkey breast sandwich
Midafternoon	Fruit	Yoghurt and nuts
Dinner	Chicken pad thai	Chicken stir-fry

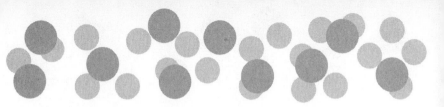

PROTEIN COUNTER		
PROTEIN SOURCE	**SERVING SIZE**	**PROTEIN PER SERVE (g)**
Beef/pork/lamb	100 g	31
Chicken/turkey	100 g	28
Seafood	100 g	23
Yoghurt	200 g	10
Baked beans	1 cup	10
Nuts	50 g	10
Milk	250 ml	9
Tofu	100 g	8
Pasta	1 cup, cooked	8
Egg	1, cooked	7
Rice	1 cup, cooked	7
Cheese	1 slice	5

Meals that contain a significant portion of protein-rich foods in addition to carbohydrates will be digested more slowly than meals or snacks that contain solely carbohydrates. Protein-rich meals and snacks will also tend to offer much more nutritionally, as they are key sources of essential nutrients including iron, zinc, calcium and omega-3 fats.

The common breakfast choices of cereal and toast with jam tend to be low in protein, as do snacks of fruit or snack bars, and lunches of plain sandwiches. Aim to include at least 20 g of protein at main meals along with 10–20 g of protein at each snack.

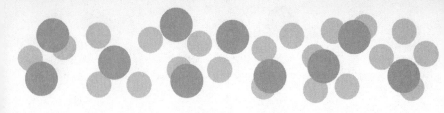

Check your good fats

'Every day we need three to four serves of good fats to enhance our cells' ability to burn body fat.'

During the 80s and 90s, much time was spent calculating the fat content of everything we ate based on the belief that a low-fat diet would surely result in a low-fat body. The truth is a little more complex than this. Effective fat metabolism (burning) is a complicated process involving a

FAT COUNTER		
FOOD	TOTAL FAT (g)	SATURATED FAT (g)
2 sausages	26	12
1 serve hot chips	25	12
2 slices cheese	13	8
200 g lean mince	14	7
½ avocado	27	6
1 glass full-cream milk	10	6
200 g Atlantic salmon	17	6
10 walnuts	21	1
1 glass low-fat milk	4	1
1 tsp olive oil	5	<1

Remember the average adult needs just 40–60 g of (predominately good) fat per day.

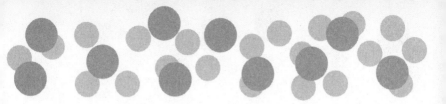

range of different types of fats that come from different foods, in different amounts. As scientists wade through the complex biochemistry, the good news for you is that there are a few key foods that you can include regularly in your diet that will help to achieve an optimal balance of the different types of fat without having to think too much at all.

Fat per gram contains 9 calories of energy. There are two types of fat; saturated and unsaturated. Saturated fat is found predominately in animal-based and processed foods, is known to increase blood cholesterol and is stored more readily than unsaturated fat. Unsaturated fat, which is found predominately in plant-based foods, including oils, nuts, seeds and avocados, as well as in oily fish (omega-3), does not increase blood cholesterol and is also more likely to be burnt off than saturated fat.

For a healthy heart and weight control, minimising your intake of saturated fat needs to be the goal for all adults. Dairy food and meat remain the greatest sources of saturated fat in our diet, which is why low-fat milk and lean cuts of meat are recommended by health professionals.

Minimising your saturated fat intake does not mean unsaturated fat can be consumed freely. The average adult needs just 40–60 g of fat in total each day. This equates to a serve of oily fish, 10 nuts, a tablespoon of avocado and a teaspoon of olive oil. So if you have been trying to lose weight for some time and are adding a whole avocado to your salad each night, it may simply be a case of too much good fat.

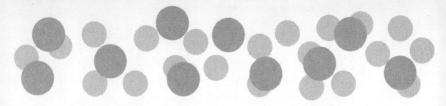

Getting your fat balance right

1   Always choose the leanest meats and low-fat dairy foods.
2   Avoid fatty sausages, salamis and processed meats.
3   Take fish oil capsules.
4   Aim to eat oily fish such as tuna, salmon (see recipe on next page) or sardines three times a week.
5   Eat a handful of nuts each day.
6   Cook with olive or canola oil.
7   Choose grain-based bread and crackers.
8   Avoid biscuits, cakes and pastries made using palm oil or hydrogenated vegetable shortening.
9   Avoid fast-food outlets that cook with lard or hydrogenated vegetable oils.

SALMON WITH VEGETABLE MASH

Vegetable mash

1 teaspoon olive oil

1 onion, finely sliced

1 small clove garlic, crushed

1 zucchini, grated

1 large carrot, grated

½ butternut pumpkin, peeled and diced

2 teaspoons low-fat olive oil spread

4 x 150 g salmon fillets, de-boned and skin removed

2 teaspoons wholegrain mustard

¼ cup low-fat sour cream

Serves 4

1 Heat oil in a pan over a medium heat, add onion and garlic. Cook for 2–3 minutes until soft. Stir in grated vegetables and cook for a further 5–8 minutes, or until vegetables are cooked.

2 Place pumpkin in a microwave-safe bowl and add a dash of water. Cover and cook on high for 5 minutes, or until tender.

3 Drain and add cooked pumpkin to vegetable mix, mashing together until smooth. Stir through olive oil spread and season with salt and pepper to taste. Set aside in a warm place until required.

4 Heat a chargrill pan over a medium-high heat. Cook salmon fillets for 3 minutes on one side. Turn over and cook for a further 1–2 minutes for medium rare or until cooked to your liking. Remove and rest for a few minutes.

5 Mix mustard and sour cream together. Top salmon fillets with a dollop of mustard cream. Serve immediately with the mash.

The importance of PUFAs

'Of all the key nutrients we need but do not get enough of, PUFAs – or long-chain polyunsaturated fats – are at the top of the list.'

As previously discussed, fat balance in the body is controlled by a number of complex metabolic pathways. It is for this reason that dietary balance never comes down to just one food or diet but rather the interplay of dietary patterns and nutrient intake, as well as our genetic response to these things. When described in relatively simple terms, there are fats that promote the health of our cells, and fats that are damaging. As the types of food we consume on a daily basis will contain a mix of the different fats, these fats compete for position in the body. Having the right ratio of the different fats is a key predictor of the health of our cells, and our body overall.

In general, Australians' intake of saturated fats is relatively high thanks to a high intake of dairy, meat, processed and fast foods. A high intake of saturated fat, especially as part of a diet in which excessive calories are consumed, is linked to increased inflammation in the body, and fat storage in the body's cells. Good fats – which include both monounsaturated fats found primarily in olive oil, peanuts, almonds and avocado and the long-chain polyunsaturated fats found in grains, seeds, walnuts and oily fish – help to balance out these fats and improve the health of our cells. While our intake of monounsaturated fats is pretty

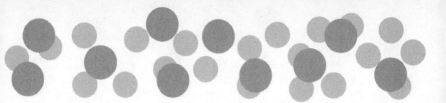

good (thanks to our love affair with olive oil and avocado), few of us get the amount of long-chain polyunsaturated fats we need to allow them to get into the cells and do their good work.

The reason for this is that natural, long-chain polyunsaturated fats are hard to find, especially if you do not eat fish. So, for anyone wanting to optimise their health, or for anyone battling autoimmune conditions such as PCOS, insulin resistance, fatty liver, thyroid issues or joint pain, here are some key foods rich in polyunsaturated fats to include in your diet to ensure you get the 10–20 g you need every day.

PUMPKIN SEEDS
Also known as pepitas, pumpkin seeds offer us a massive dose of these special fats. Just 30 g of pepitas offer almost 7 g of long-chain fats, or a third of our daily requirement.

WALNUTS
All nuts are good for us but walnuts, in particular, pack a massive punch when it comes to omega 3. Just 10–12 walnuts offer more than 14 g of long-chain fats.

SALMON
It is not for nothing that dietitians regularly cite salmon as one of the favourite superfoods – one of the few naturally occurring sources of the powerful long-chain fatty acids EPA and DHA, a 100 g serve of salmon will give you at least 4 g of these fats. And while plant sources of these fats

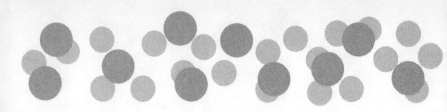

are still good choices nutritionally (they convert to the longer chain EPA and DHA), oily fish remains the richest source of DHA and EPA.

SOY LINSEED BREAD

While all grain bread is a good choice, it is specifically the mix of soy and linseed that gives soy linseed bread its 4 g of polyunsaturated fats per serve.

CHIA

Another super seed that offers more than 3 g of long-chain fats per tablespoon.

SARDINES

There are few commonly consumed fish in Australia that are naturally rich in omega 3 fats but sardines are one of them. They contain 3 g of polyunsaturated fats per serve.

PECANS

If walnuts are not your thing, a 30 g serve of approximately 20 pecans will offer more than 7 g of long-chain fats.

SESAME SEEDS

Rich in long-chain fats with more than 3 g of polyunsaturated fats per serve.

Avoid the diet food

'I will never be convinced that artificial sweetener is a better option than sugar.'

It all sounds so great – diet soft drink, diet yoghurt, diet chocolate, even diet desserts. Finally we can have all of our favourite foods for fewer calories and less chance of weight gain. Unfortunately, as is the case with all things in life, if it seems too good to be true, it usually is.

Diet foods have lower calories than the regular varieties as they have been sweetened using artificial sweeteners. Artificial sweeteners, including sucralose, saccharin and aspartame, are synthetically developed substances that have a similar chemical structure to various sugars but are up to 500 times sweeter. Such intense sweetness means that only small amounts of these artificial substances are required to make a food taste even sweeter than the original food, with fewer calories.

Initially nutritionists reported a number of benefits of consuming less sugar and calories via artificially sweetened food. But emerging evidence suggests that consuming large volumes of these foods may actually prime the brain to crave increasingly sweeter food. It also appears that the brain may not optimally regulate the calories consumed in products containing sweeteners, such as diet yoghurt, as they often lack the mouth-feel of foods with a regular carbohydrate profile. This means we don't feel as satisfied after eating such products and are likely to eat more.

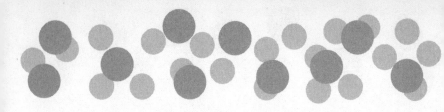

While swapping to a diet product, especially in the case of soft drink, is a better alternative than choosing the full-sugar version, the truth is that neither product is a healthy component of anyone's diet. While there is nothing wrong with an occasional diet drink, they should not be replacing water as a regular fluid choice.

For those attempting to get back in touch with their body's natural hunger and fullness signals, eliminating the use of sweetener in hot beverages, yoghurts and desserts is a good starting point. Instead of allowing yourself to eat more because it's 'diet', try eating smaller amounts of non-diet foods you enjoy, such as low-fat yoghurt or your favourite dessert. You will find that eating the real thing satisfies you after a smaller amount and you will enjoy it much more. A small amount of sugar that you gradually reduce in your favourite tea or coffee is also a much better option than dosing yourself up on exceptionally sweet drinks all day.

No matter how much we engineer our foods to be lower in calories or richer in flavour, the more natural and clean our food is, the better it will be for us.

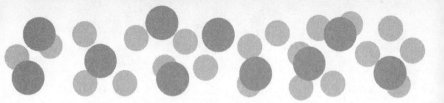

'Tis sugar, 'tis sugar, 'tis sugar

'If it looks like sugar and tastes like sugar, it's probably sugar.'

Nothing makes a scientist laugh more than seeing low-sugar diets packed with dried fruit, rice malt syrup, dextrose and coconut sugar. While it is often claimed that these are 'better' sugars, one can argue that when you take a closer look at the chemistry, these are still all sugars – sugars that will contribute to weight gain, hormonal imbalance and cravings if overconsumed. So just in case you think you are aboard the anti-sugar band wagon but your recipes are still full of rice malt syrup and coconut sugar, it may pay to take a closer look at what sugar actually is and what it is not.

SIMPLE SUGARS
Naturally occurring simple sugars contain 4 calories per gram. On the whole, simple sugars offer 'empty' calories: meaning they offer little nutritionally other than extra energy and for this reason should be consumed in small amounts.

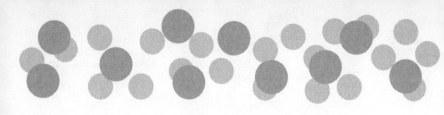

HONEY

Often chosen as a natural alternative to white sugar thanks to its antibacterial properties, honey still contains 5 g of total sugars and 19 calories per teaspoon.

RICE MALT SYRUP

Often considered much better for you than sugar, the harsh truth is that rice malt syrup is a refined sugar that is produced by cooking rice flour or starch with enzymes. With a GI of 98 (white bread = 100), its supremacy as an alternative to table sugar is highly questionable. The sugar mix of rice malt syrup is 3 per cent glucose, 45 per cent maltose and 52 per cent maltotriose. While it may be fructose free, it is not concentrated calorie free.

AGAVE

Agave is sourced from the agave plant, which is found in Mexico. It is popular as it appears to have a more moderate effect on blood glucose levels than refined sugar. Agave has slightly less total sugar and calories per serve than regular sugar, but is roughly 1½ times sweeter than sugar so you can use less of it. It is also high in fructose, which can cause gut distress for those who are sensitive.

RAW SUGAR

Often thought of as a better option nutritionally than white sugar, raw sugar is less refined than white sugar. It still contains the same number of calories per serve as white or brown sugar.

NATURAL SWEETENERS

These are generally sourced from plants and taste as sweet, or sweeter than, sugar minus the calories. However, as mentioned in the previous chapter, whilst the calories in many of these sweeteners may be negligible, there is some evidence to show that consuming exceptionally sweet foods may actually program the brain to seek out sweeter food. For this reason, while natural sweeteners may appear to be a good option, they should certainly not be used in unlimited quantities.

STEVIA

Sourced from a South African plant, stevia is 200–300 times sweeter than sugar and is now used frequently in yoghurts, cordials and soft drinks. Often referred to as the best natural sweetener available, it can also be used effectively in baking to reduce the sugar content of a recipe.

NATVIA

Combines stevia with erithrytol (a sugar alcohol) to offer another plant-based sweetener that seeks to eliminate the sometimes-bitter aftertaste experienced with stevia. Ideally any sweetener should be used in small amounts due to its intensely sweet flavour and Natvia, in particular, is best used in tea and coffee.

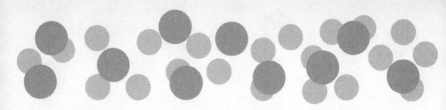

SUGAR ALCOHOLS

Commonly listed as mannitol, sorbitol and xylitol on ingredient lists, sugar alcohols are carbohydrates naturally found in some fruit and vegetables. They are only partially broken down in the digestive track and as such offer up to 40 per cent fewer calories than sugar. While sugar alcohols are a natural sweetener that can be used in baking and to sweeten drinks, for people with sensitive stomachs, or who report symptoms of irritable bowel syndrome, sugar alcohols can cause bloating, diarrhoea and gas.

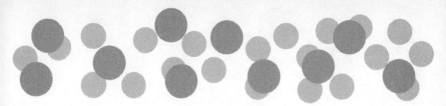

CHILLI STEAK

2 x 200 g rib-eye steaks

olive oil cooking spray

100 g baby spinach leaves

2 medium tomatoes,
halved, then sliced

50 g low-fat fetta,
crumbled

15 walnuts

½ red chilli, finely chopped

extra-virgin olive oil to serve

balsamic vinegar to serve

1 Heat a barbecue plate or chargrill pan to high. Spray the steaks with cooking spray, then cook for 3–4 minutes on each side for medium, or until done to your liking. Remove from the heat and rest, covered, in a warm place for 5 minutes.

2 In a bowl, gently toss together the spinach, tomato, fetta, walnuts and chilli. Mix oil and vinegar, then drizzle over steak to serve.

Serves 2

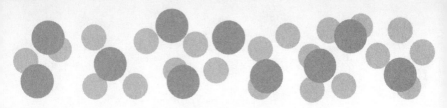

What are you drinking?

'Liquid calories are easily consumed and rarely counted. Water should be the primary fluid of choice for us all.'

Sweetened drinks are a recipe for disaster when it comes to our weight control. Liquid calories can add up quickly, often without us realising, and offer very little nutritionally.

FRUIT JUICE

Freshly squeezed fruit juice seems to epitomise good health. But while fresh fruit is a nutrient-dense snack choice packed with fibre, vitamins and minerals, the concentration of fresh fruit juice means it can be a calorie-dense fluid, without the fibre and satiating properties of fresh fruit. Always choose 100 per cent fruit juice, stick to small servings (200 ml) and limit your intake to one serve a day to avoid a calorie overload. Better still, try vegetable juices, which contain a third of the calories.

TEA

Tea is a rich source of antioxidants, and evidence suggests drinking a cup of strong green tea after meals slightly increases metabolic rate. Naturally, all types of tea are best consumed without sugar.

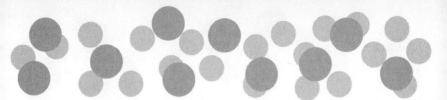

VITAMIN WATER

Vitamin waters have experienced a recent resurgence courtesy of powerful marketing campaigns promising attractive results such as 'vitality' and 'energy'. While these rather expensive waters do contain added vitamins, the reality is that these vitamins are rarely lacking in the average adult's diet. As they can contain up to 6 teaspoons of sugar per bottle, it's probably best to save your money and get your vitamins from fresh fruit and vegetables instead.

SPORTS DRINK

A specially formulated mix of rapidly absorbed carbohydrates and minerals, sports drinks help athletes in their recovery and rehydration after competition. While sports drinks play a role in high-level sport, for those training for less than an hour a day they are generally not necessary.

SOFT DRINK

With up to 9 teaspoons of sugar per 375 ml can, in addition to a number of colours and preservatives, soft drink is a calorie-dense, nutrient-poor liquid choice. If you choose to purchase diet varieties, it is useful to be aware that some of the additives used in these drinks are considered so harmful in some parts of the world that they have been banned. (See 'Avoid the diet food' for more information.)

CORDIAL

Cordial, like soft drink, is a nutrient-poor, high-calorie liquid choice and needs to be limited, for both adults and children.

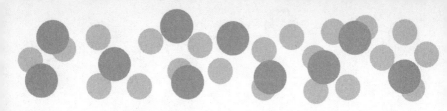

WINE

There is evidence to show that a glass of red wine a night can help to increase the good cholesterol in the bloodstream, but these results are based on drinking just 1 standard-sized glass, not a goblet.

WHAT'S IN YOUR FAVOURITE DRINKS?		
STANDARD SERVES	CALORIES	SUGAR
Regular fruit smoothie (650 ml)	360	6
Grande caramel latte (450 ml)	310	8
Cola drink (600 ml)	240	13
Sports drink (600 ml)	185	9
Large glass of wine (240 ml)	170	–
Regular beer (285 ml)	130	–
Low-fat smoothie (350 ml)	120	4
Vitamin water (500 ml)	110	4
Light beer (285 ml)	102	–
Standard glass of wine (120 ml)	85	–
Green tea (200 ml)	1	–

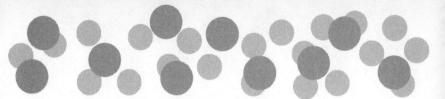

BEER

Beer doesn't offer the potential health benefits of spirits and red wine, but if it's still your drink of choice, you can significantly reduce your caloric intake by choosing low-carb, low-alcohol varieties. Remember it is recommended adults consume no more than 2 standard drinks a day with at least 2 alcohol-free days a week.

SPRITS

Spirits, like red wine, contain powerful antioxidants that appear to help increase the levels of good cholesterol in the bloodstream. Spirits do not tend to be overconsumed to the extent that wine and beer are, which can help to control calorie intake. The most important thing in relation to spirits is to watch your mixers – stick to soda water, diet soft drinks or ice to help lower your total caloric intake.

WATER

Water should be the main fluid of choice for all of us and if you are not drinking 1.5–2 litres a day, you are not drinking enough. Not only does keeping hydrated help us (and our skin) to look and feel better, it helps to prevent fatigue, bloating and constipation.

Count the coffees

'If coffee contains milk and sugar, it's a snack.'

We all love our coffee but unless you enjoy it black, it has to be counted as food. If you are enjoying 2–3 coffees with milk and/or sugar before 9 am, you have basically been eating for 3 hours and that is why you are not losing weight.

Some people would sacrifice almost anything rather than give up their daily skim cappuccino. There is nothing wrong with coffee per se, in fact, if consumed in the right amounts, coffee has a number of health benefits, including reduced blood pressure and blood fats, and can reduce your risk of developing a number of diseases including some types of cancer. The key thing to know is that the way we drink our coffee and how many times a day we do is of crucial importance when it comes to weight control.

While a long black contains as few as 2 calories and little to no carbohydrates, a regular latte contains up to 200 calories, with another 15 for every teaspoon of sugar or syrup you add. In fact, if you enjoy two or three of these coffees daily, you are effectively adding an extra 3–4 kg of body weight over the course of a year.

The best way to enjoy your coffee is with a meal or as a snack – not as an extra. The body needs at least 2–3 hours in between meals without any

YOUR FAVOURITE BREW	
COFFEE	**CALORIES***
Large flat white	220
Large low-fat latte	130
Small flat white	120
Small latte	120
Large low-fat cappuccino	100
Small low-fat latte	70
Small low-fat flat white	70
Small low-fat cappuccino	60

*Remember add an extra 15 calories for every teaspoon of sugar or syrup you add to your favourite brew.

food stimulus and this includes milk and sugar. Black tea or coffee is the best option in between meals. The other important thing to remember with coffee is that no-one needs the large size. A regular size is more than enough, for all of us.

For those who rely on coffee and drink 4 or more cups a day, it may be useful to remember that coffee is a stimulant, increasing central nervous system activity. Relying on such stimulation may mean that there are underlying issues with your diet or lifestyle that need to be addressed. Aim for no more than 3–4 cups of coffee each day and drink more water or herbal tea instead. If you know you need to cut back, it is also important that you wean yourself off gradually so you don't induce the side effects of caffeine withdrawal.

What's in your coffee?

Flat white A shot of espresso with two parts steamed milk, 120 calories and 7 g of fat. Swapping to skim milk will reduce this to 70 calories and almost no fat, although some fat may help to keep you full.

Latte A shot of espresso with two parts frothed milk. Similar nutritional content to a full fat flat white with 120 calories and 7 g of fat with just 70 calories and no fat for a small sized skim milk serve. A good source of calcium.

Cappuccino A shot of espresso with a third milk and a third froth; slightly lower in calories than a latte or flat white with 110 calories and 6 g of fat with full cream milk. Slightly lower calcium content than both a latte and flat white as it contains slightly less milk.

Macchiato A shot of coffee with a dash of milk – will contain just 13 or 18 calories depending on whether the milk added is skim or full cream. The risk with this form of coffee is that many people will add sugar, which will add 15 calories per teaspoon.

Piccolo latte A mini version of a latte with just 45 calories if with full cream milk or 25 if you go for skim. A great option for those who enjoy the taste of coffee but do not need the extra calories.

Mocha A latte with an extra shot of chocolate syrup added. Contains significantly more carbohydrates and calories than the average coffee, with 160 calories and 6 g of fat in the full cream version or 100 calories and virtually no fat in the skim milk version.

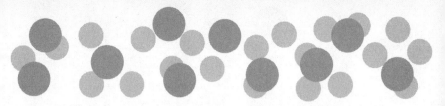

Soy latte A latte made using soy milk instead of dairy milk. Many soy-based coffees are made using full fat soy milk, which can bump up the calories. A small will give you 3 g of fat and 80 calories.

Chai latte While it may appear to be a 'healthy choice' the good old chai powder found at many coffee shops is packed with sugar. A small chai will give you 130 calories and 2 g of fat but an extra 20 g (4 teaspoons) of sugar.

Long black Next to the macchiato, the long black is a favourite for coffee lovers with a shot of espresso slightly diluted with hot water. At 4 calories per serve, minus any milk or sugar, one or two of these will will be good for both your love of coffee and your diet.

Bulletproof coffee Popular with paleo fans, bulletproof coffee combines black coffee with butter and a tablespoon of oil and is generally used as part of a dietary regime that significantly increases your fat intake at the expense of carbs. Offering 50 g of fat and almost 480 calories per serve, this breakfast option would almost certainly lead to weight gain unless consumed as a part of a very specific diet.

Almond milk coffee Swapping both regular milk and soy for almond is becoming increasingly popular. While almond milk may appear exceptionally low in calories, it is also very low in nutrients including protein and calcium; often contains added oil and sugars and is generally only a suggested option for individuals unable to tolerate dairy or soy, rather than a better option nutritionally.

* All values are based on a small serve = 220 ml.

Go 1 month alcohol-free

'An alcohol-free period in the early stages of weight loss is vital.'

Some clients enjoy cheese, others chocolate and others would rather eat bread and water if it meant they could still enjoy a glass of wine at the end of each day.

Alcohol, the fourth most energy-containing nutrient after carbohydrate, protein and fat, contains 7 calories of energy per gram, only slightly less than fat, which contains 9 calories per gram. Not only is alcohol relatively high in energy, it is recognised as a toxin by the body and therefore digested before the other three nutrients. This means if you eat when you drink, the body will be so busy burning up the alcohol that it is less likely to get to the food, which is why alcohol and weight gain go hand in hand.

While a small glass of wine contains the same amount of calories as a few pieces of chocolate, the jumbo-sized glasses it is often served in can contain three times this amount. Low-carb and reduced-alcohol varieties are slightly better options, but such a benefit is quickly lost when three or four times the recommended number of drinks is consumed. For most people, one or two standard drinks a night will not cause weight gain per se, the danger comes from the foods we commonly enjoy with them, such as cheese, dips and potato chips.

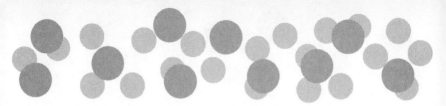

In theory, if your caloric intake is below your energy output, even with the inclusion of a glass or two you should still lose weight. Unfortunately in my experience, this is not the case. Perhaps it is because we eat more when we drink, or that we commonly drink at night, or because we have goblet-sized wine glasses. Whatever the reason, if you are serious about weight loss and are a regular drinker, making a decision to go alcohol-free for a month may be the kickstart you need to see a change in the scales, to discover how much you really have been drinking, and to consider if you are really drinking for enjoyment or out of habit.

COMMONLY CONSUMED ALCOHOL	
DRINK	CALORIES
2 regular beers	285
Pre-mixed spirit	165
Large (typical) glass of wine	155
Bourbon and cola	120
Low-carb beer	105
Small glass of wine	90
Small glass of champagne	85
Glass of low-alcohol wine	75
Bourbon and diet cola	70
Remember we need a total of 1500—2000 calories on average per day.	

To snack or not to snack?

'There is nothing wrong with enjoying a small snack when you are hungry, but often a small snack becomes a meal without us noticing – that is the issue.'

Snacks were once considered extremely important to keep the metabolism pumping. Unfortunately, what was once considered a small snack (a piece of fruit or a coffee) is now more likely a small meal's worth of calories as we overdo the muffins, snack bars and smoothies. These days we tend to eat far too much, too often, which inevitably leads to weight gain. So, do you need to snack and if so, what are your best choices?

The average human needs to eat every 3–5 hours – the range is wide depending on age, gender, lifestyle and activity levels. Traditionally eating three square meals each day, say breakfast by 8 am, lunch at 12 and dinner at 6 pm, meant there was little need to snack, with the exception of an occasional piece of fruit in between meals. Fast-forward 50 or 60 years and snacking is promoted, both to keep our energy and concentration levels up in between meals and to break up the day.

If you consider the average workday, where breakfast is consumed early, it is plausible that you might be hungry midmorning (around 10 am

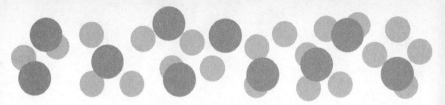

or 11 am) for something to tie you over until lunchtime. Here, just a 100–200 calorie snack of a milk coffee, banana or some cheese and crackers is more than enough to get through another hour or two until lunch. Often we enjoy a milk coffee or juice along with something to eat, when really we only need one or the other.

On the other hand, if you do not eat breakfast until 8 or 9 in the morning, you are better to have an early lunch than eat a snack within an hour or two of lunch. Moving into the afternoon, again the need to snack will depend on the size and timing of your lunch, and how long it will be until your evening meal. If you consume your lunch by 1 pm and will not be eating dinner until 6 or 7 pm, again you will most likely need a reasonable 200–300 calorie snack around 4 pm to keep your hunger controlled until dinner time. Options that include a mix of both carbohydrates for energy as well as protein to help control your appetite are good choices. A piece of fruit teamed with some Greek yoghurt, a nut-based snack bar or some crackers with tuna or cheese are all filling, nutritionally balanced options.

A handy way to consider snacking is that it needs to keep you full for at least a couple of hours. For this reason, plain biscuits, lollies, chocolates and processed snack bars are never the best choice.

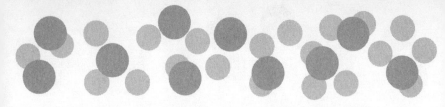

Top 10 snack choices

1 Nut-based snack bar

2 4 grain crackers with cheese

3 Small skim latte

4 100 g thick yoghurt and berries

5 2 corn crackers with cottage cheese

6 ½ cup edamame beans

7 2 cups popcorn

8 Mini protein bar and a piece of fruit

9 2 rye crackers with goat's cheese and tomato

10 Small hommus with vegetables

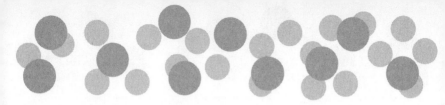

CHOC PEPPERMINT BLISS BALLS

1 cup almond meal

¼ cup coconut flour

1 tablespoon cocoa powder

½ scoop vanilla protein powder
(use vegan protein powder
if needed)

¼ cup water

¼ teaspoon stevia

pinch of salt

¼ teaspoon vanilla extract

few drops peppermint extract

1 tablespoon honey

¼ cup almonds, crushed

Serves 5

1 Mix almond meal, coconut flour and cocoa in a large bowl.

2 In a small bowl mix protein powder, water, stevia, salt and vanilla extract. Add to the dry ingredients a bit at a time whilst mixing.

3 Once combined, add the peppermint extract and honey.

4 Use heaped tablespoons of the mixture to roll into balls and then roll in extra coconut flour and crushed almonds.

5 Refrigerate for an hour until set and either keep in the fridge or an airtight container.

Nuts once a day

'Remember a serve of nuts is just ten, not half the packet.'

Yes, it is true – nuts are very good for us. In fact, a 30 g serving per day is actually linked to weight control long-term. However, knowing that nuts are good for us does not mean we can eat them in unlimited volumes. Nuts, like seeds and grains, are relatively high in fat, but the good news is that this fat is predominately unsaturated, the type of fat that contributes to optimal cell health, helps to regulate a number of hormones and improves good cholesterol levels. Often dieters will keep their total fat intake low and forget the crucial importance of good fats that actually optimise fat metabolism. A serve of 10 nuts each day ensures that we are getting a good dose of poly- and mono-unsaturated fat, protein, fibre and vitamin E.

Aim for a nut-based snack late in the afternoon. Not only will this help to ward off the pre-dinner munchies, but the low-carb content will help to taper your fuel intake towards the second half of the day, which is conducive to weight control.

When it comes to which type, walnuts stand out as the clear winner. Walnuts are known as a 'superfood' as they contain exceptionally high amounts of the long-chain poly-unsaturated fats. For this reason,

individuals with high cholesterol can reap many benefits of adding
10 walnuts a day to their diet. The other favourites – peanuts, almonds
and cashews – are much higher in mono-unsaturated fats. Their health
benefits also tend to be present in a number of commonly eaten foods,
including avocado and olive oil.

When purchasing nuts, remember that freshness matters. The fresher
the nut, the better its nutrient levels will be. Purchasing your nuts from
growers' markets or retailers who have a high turnover will help ensure
that you have fresher, better tasting nuts. But remember portion control is
key. If you buy your nuts in large bags, repackage them immediately into
portion controlled serves.

HOW MUCH FAT IS IN NUTS?				
SERVE OF 10	TOTAL FAT (g)	POLY FAT (g)	MONO FAT (g)	SAT FAT (g)
Walnuts	21	15	4	1
Macadamias	15	<1	12	2
Almonds	7	2	4	<1
Cashews	7	1	5	1
Peanuts	4	1	2	1

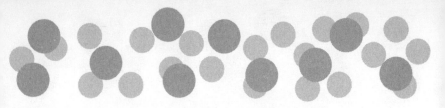

SPRING LAMB WITH WALNUTS & BEETROOT

4 beetroots, peeled and cubed

2 tablespoons garlic infused oil

4 tablespoons balsamic vinegar

3 sprigs rosemary, destemmed

8 lamb cutlets, lean

100 g walnut, roughly chopped

160 g spinach

160 g rocket

Serves 4

1 Preheat the oven to 200°C.

2 Place the beetroot on a baking tray, drizzle with half the oil, the balsamic vinegar and season with salt and pepper. Cook in the oven for 30 minutes.

3 Combine the rest of the oil with the rosemary and a dash of salt and pepper. Rub over the lamb chops.

4 Heat a non-stick pan over medium to high heat. Add the lamb and cook for 2–4 minutes on each side.

5 Roughly chop the walnuts.

6 Removing the beetroot from the oven, mix through the baby spinach, rocket and walnuts.

7 Divide the salad between plates and serve with the lamb cutlets.

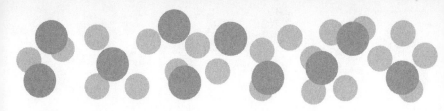

Never leave the house without two vegetables

'Remember if it's in front of you, you will eat it.'

It may seem like a strange suggestion but always having a vegetable-based snack with you – whether it be a carrot, some celery sticks or baby tomatoes – means you are more likely to get the number of vegetable serves that you need each day and also always have a filling snack on hand.

Many of us eat too many calories simply because we do not eat enough of the low-calorie foods to bulk up our diet and keep us full. Meals and snacks we choose on the run often contain a small volume of vegetable bulk, but it is exceptionally easy to add. Munching on a carrot or celery, or adding tomatoes or rocket to crackers will bulk up your diet and leave you craving fewer snacks.

The 'two vegetables' rule will become as easy as remembering to grab your keys as you leave the house. You will need to purchase larger volumes of vegetables and salad each week so you always have supplies on hand. Remember, if it's in front of you, you will eat it.

Know the best treats

'There is nothing wrong with eating some chocolate – it's eating the whole block that brings things undone.'

Chips, chocolate, cheese and cakes – imagine how easy it would be to manage your weight without the 4 Cs? The danger with these tasty treats is that they are not only very high in fat, but they are also very easy to overeat. A block of chocolate while watching TV, a 200 g packet of chips at a barbecue, a round of brie with a glass of wine and you have consumed a massive amount of both fat and calories.

There is growing evidence that the complex mix of sugar and fat found in chocolate, ice-cream, cakes and pastries may actually prime the brain to seek more and more of this type of food. Such intense flavours light up reward centres in the brain, which over time encourages the brain to look for such stimulation again. Eating these foods reinforces the brain's cravings rather than satisfying them.

We have often been programmed from an early age to strongly desire the 4 Cs. Many of us will have powerful memories of parents hiding treat foods, rewarding good behaviour with chocolate and only having chips and cake on special occasions. These restrictions program our brain to seek reward from these foods and strongly desire what we have not been freely allowed. This reaction tends to be worse the more restricted the food has been. This is why some children will overeat at birthday

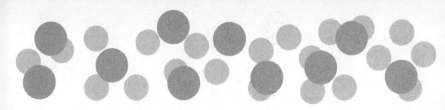

parties – they have been constantly deprived of certain foods so have not learnt how to regulate their intake when they are readily available.

Ideally by the time we reach adulthood, we would have learnt to manage ourselves around these types of food. We would be able to keep a block of chocolate in the fridge but only enjoy a few pieces at a time, or not eat the whole packet of biscuits simply because they are there. However, for many of us, this early programming is too strong, and limiting our exposure to these tempting treats is the best way to control ourselves until we break the habit.

If you struggle with portions, buying blocks of chocolate or large tubs of ice-cream is dangerous. Buy portion-controlled options only, or buy them only as you need them if you really struggle. Incorporating your favourite foods into your daily diet is the best way to develop a sustainable model of eating without negative effects on weight control.

KNOWING THE 4 Cs		
TREATS	CALORIES	FAT (g)
250 g block of chocolate	1300	68
1 slice of mud cake	310	17
1 slice of banana bread	300	20
50 g packet of potato chips	260	17
A few pieces of chocolate	150	8
¼ round of brie	100	9
30 g fetta cheese	80	7

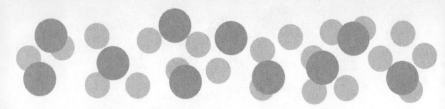

Low-calorie treats

2 squares of dark chocolate

1 individually wrapped chocolate

1 chocolate biscuit

1 low-fat hot chocolate

1 low-fat ice-cream on a stick

1 mango ice-cream bar

1 muesli cookie

2 rye crackers and 1 slice of low-fat cheese

2 corn crackers with low-fat cream cheese

2 tablespoons of thick yoghurt with berries

Breakfast success

*'There is no point even trying to lose weight unless
you are eating a protein-rich breakfast before 8 am.'*

Despite strong evidence that breakfast helps boost metabolic rate and
fat loss, there are still many of us who do not get our first meal of the day
right. Choosing high-GI breakfast options such as sugary cereals, Turkish
toast or bagels, or skipping breakfast altogether can leave you more likely
to overeat during the rest of the day and ultimately lead to long-term
weight gain. Breakfast skippers often claim they feel ill if they eat early.
This is merely a result of programming the body not to look for food until
much later in the day and will subside once you start slowly reintroducing
small breakfasts. The good news is that for even those completely turned
off by the thought of cereal and milk, a healthy breakfast can be simple
once you know a few tricks of food digestion and metabolism.

The first thing to keep in mind is that the body's digestive hormones are
programmed according to a 24-hour circadian rhythm. This means that
after an overnight fast of 8–12 hours without food, the body is ready
to refuel with energy from carbohydrates. Failing to refuel for an extra
3–4 hours by putting off breakfast until 10 or 11am slows the metabolic
rate as the body senses starvation and acts to conserve energy. It even

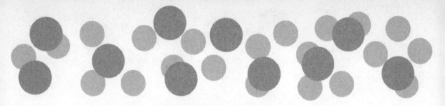

seems the bigger the better when it comes to our breakfast choices. A recent paper published in the *International Journal of Obesity* found that individuals on a weight-loss diet lost twice as much body fat when they consumed half of their daily calories at breakfast.

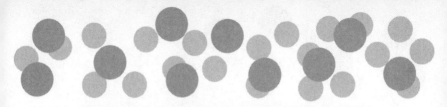

Top 10 breakfast options

1 1–2 poached eggs on 1–2 slices of wholegrain toast
2 130 g tin of baked beans on 1 slice of wholegrain toast
3 ⅓ cup oats + 1 cup low-fat milk
4 Protein shake or liquid-meal drink
5 Egg breakfast wrap
6 ⅓ cup muesli + thick yoghurt + fruit
7 ¾ cup wholegrain breakfast cereal + low-fat milk
8 Protein bar or breakfast bar
9 Low-fat latte + 1 piece of fruit
10 Smoked salmon on 1–2 slices of wholegrain toast

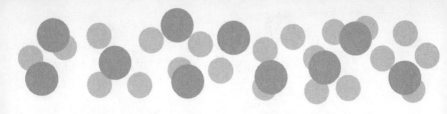

THE MOST COMMON BREAKFAST MISTAKES

Are you eating breakfast too late? As a general rule of thumb, the earlier you enjoy your breakfast, the better it will be for your metabolism. It is commonly thought that delaying hunger until later in the morning or waiting until after a workout will optimise fat burning; but the truth is that you will train more effectively if you have something small beforehand and then have a more substantial meal after training. Light breakfast options include a slice of wholegrain toast with peanut butter, a couple of crackers with cheese, or a banana. This is all you need to get your metabolism going. Ideally, you will back this up with a high protein breakfast such as eggs, protein pancakes or Greek yoghurt and fruit later in the morning.

Are you getting the right nutrient mix? An ideal balance of wholegrain, low glycaemic index carbohydrates and 15–20 g of protein at breakfast will ensure that you have well controlled blood glucose levels, energy throughout the morning, and keep you full and satisfied for at least 3–4 hours (ideally until lunchtime). Choices that have a high carbohydrate load relative to protein such as toast with a spread, large serves of cereal, raisin toast, muffins and Turkish breads leave you vulnerable to high insulin levels and hunger throughout the morning. Better choices include eggs on toast, a protein and banana smoothie or Greek yoghurt with fruit.

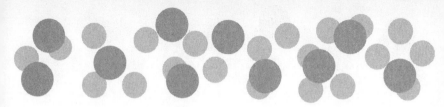

Are you forgetting the coffee? Flat whites, cappuccinos, soy mochas and chai lattes all contain calories and sugars (generally from the lactose naturally found in milk). These need to be considered as part of a meal, not an insignificant extra. For any coffee that contains a significant amount of milk, consider it as equal in calories to a slice of toast. If you are watching your total calorie and/or sugar intake, consider swapping to black coffee or tea to cut out some of these extra calories.

Are you overindulging in a café breakfast? For city workers, or anyone who has a great café close to home or work that offers coffee and toast for a cheap price, it can be hard to resist a daily café treat. Unfortunately, the types of breakfast options served at cafés rarely complement our dietary goals. Large slices of Turkish toast slathered in butter; sandwiches with cheese and fatty meats; oversized muffins; and thick sugary yoghurt and granola can equate to 600–800 breakfast calories – more than double what the average person needs. Save the café breakfasts for weekends or special occasions, or at least look for lighter options such as an omelette with one thin slice of toast, mini breakfast wraps or Greek yoghurt and fruit.

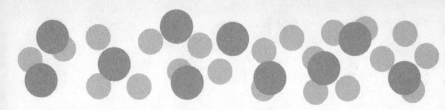

No time to prepare a healthy breakfast Not having enough time to prepare a nutritionally balanced breakfast is one of the most common reasons we end up overindulging with the muffins and fried breakfasts we pick up on the run. The easiest way to take control of these poor breakfast choices is to get into a habit of preparing a nutritionally balanced breakfast the night before. Homemade Bircher muesli with oats, banana and Greek yoghurt; breakfast wraps with lean meat and cheese; or hard-boiled eggs or a frittata can all be prepared the night before and then enjoyed the next day.

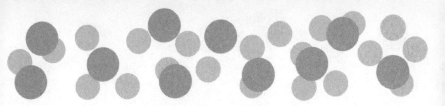

SMOKED SALMON FRITTATA MUFFINS

6 eggs

1 medium sweet potato, peeled, diced into 1 cm cubes

4 medium mushrooms, diced

1 cup baby spinach leaves, shredded

4 slices (100 g) smoked salmon, diced

olive oil spray

cracked black pepper, to taste

Serves 4

1 Preheat oven to 180–200°C and lightly spray an 8-cup muffin tray with the olive oil spray.

2 Whisk eggs and set aside.

3 Microwave the sweet potato until just tender (remember to add some water to your microwave-safe bowl first). Drain well.

4 Evenly distribute the mushrooms, spinach, sweet potato and smoked salmon amongst the muffin cups. Pour over the beaten egg. Season with pepper.

5 Cook in the preheated oven for 15–20 minutes or until cooked through.

Get your lunch balance right

'If you are craving sugar at 4 pm, you haven't eaten properly at lunchtime.'

After years of reading nutrition information you know that breakfast is important, and that you need to eat more vegetables. You also know that a tuna salad is a good choice for lunch – or is it? What we choose for lunch as well as the time we eat it can have a big impact on the way we eat and feel for the remainder of the day. This is a nutrition area surprisingly overlooked, particularly by busy people. Getting the balance right is very easy, as is preparing a tasty yet nutritious lunch which may be slightly more appealing than your usual – but rather dull – tuna and salad.

SOME GOOD-QUALITY CARBS

The first component of a nutritionally balanced lunch is a serve of low-GI carbs. For all the carb-phobics out there who try and keep their intake as low as possible, remember that carbs are the main fuel for the muscle. Choosing to starve your muscles of carbs throughout the day is more likely to leave you craving them later in the afternoon. A much better approach is to include a serve of low-GI carbs at lunch and then keep your intake of energy-dense carbs such as biscuits, cakes and bread lighter during the second half of the day.

Tinned beans or corn, wholemeal pasta or brown rice, wholegrain crackers or 1–2 slices of dense grain, flat or sourdough bread are all good

lunch choices. Naturally, people who are more active require more carbs throughout the day than those who are less active. As a rough guide, a female who exercises for an hour each day will need roughly 1 cup of rice or pasta or 2 slices of bread. A more active, large male will require more; a more sedentary person less.

A SERVE OF NUTRIENT-RICH PROTEIN

A couple of slices of ham is not enough. We need a good-sized serve of lean protein included in our lunch choice to help avoid the 3–4 pm munchies. Tins of tuna or salmon, a palm-sized piece of chicken breast or lean red meat, an egg or tofu are nutrient-rich options that will ensure your salad, sandwich or sushi will keep you full throughout the afternoon. Always keep a couple of tins of tuna handy in your desk drawer to add to salads or vegetables, or plan ahead and make enough dinner to give you tasty leftovers if you struggle with eating protein in your lunch.

MORE VEGETABLES OR SALAD THAN YOU THINK!

The most common mistake healthy eaters make is forgetting how much salad and vegetable bulk they need in their lunch. A few lettuce leaves or tomato slices is not enough – ideally you need at least 3–4 different vegetables with your lunch to give you the fibre, vitamins, minerals and bulk that will keep you full throughout the afternoon. Carry hard vegetables such as carrots and celery with you to munch on, or prepare an extra green salad the night before to enjoy with your regular sandwich, soup or sushi.

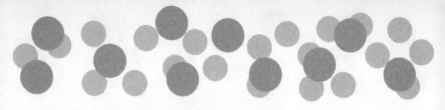

WORST LUNCH CHOICES		
FOOD CHOICE	CALORIES	FAT (g)
Burger and fries	880	40
Pad thai	810	46
Chicken and avocado on Turkish bread	760	54
Quiche	475	30
Stir-fry chicken and rice	475	30
Pesto chicken salad	475	35

TOP LUNCH CHOICES		
FOOD CHOICE	CALORIES	FAT (g)
Leftover pasta with meat and vegetable sauce	330	7
2 tuna sushi rolls	330	6
Wholegrain crackers with salmon and rocket	285	6
Chicken and salad wrap	285	6
Frittata and salad	285	7
Tuna, beans and salad	240	7

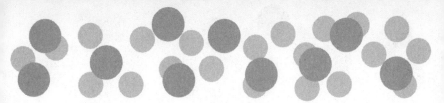

The best healthy lunch choices on the go

'While it is harder to make healthy choices away from home, it is not impossible.'

When you take a quick scan around the local food court, or at the menu at your local café, chances are the popular lunchtime choices of a schnitzel sandwich, Caesar salad or creamy salad are not all that healthy. So what can you pick up at lunchtime when you are in a rush?

A HEALTHY WRAP

Making your own wrap or sandwich will always be a better option nutritionally than buying a pre-made option. Lean, protein-rich options such as turkey, chicken, tuna or egg with plenty of salad are the way to go. Generally speaking, wraps will have fewer carbs and calories than thick slices of sourdough and Turkish bread. A regular wrap with chicken breast and salad contains between 350–400 calories and will help to keep you full for several hours. In cases where the wraps are large, another option is to eat half as an early lunch and the other half for afternoon tea.

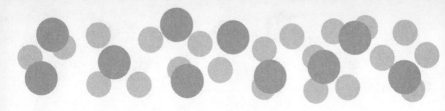

Turkey or chicken salad wrap
Total calories = 400–500
Total fat = 10–15 g
Total carbs = 35–40 g
Total sugars = 2 g

CHICKEN STRIPS

If you must make a fast food choice, the good news is that the chicken strips offered at a number of fast food chains can be a strong choice nutritionally. With <10–15 g of total fat per serve they can make a balanced lunch choice, especially if teamed with salad (as opposed to fries and a soft drink).

4 chicken strips and salad
Total calories = 360
Total fat = 12 g
Total carbs = 10 g
Total sugars = 4 g

MEXICAN BOWL

Mexican cuisine in food courts is a great choice nutritionally if you opt for the naked bowls they offer. Basically, a burrito minus the wrap, served in a bowl: a naked burrito bowl is a protein- and vegetable-rich lunch choice and can be relatively low in fat if you go easy on the sour cream, cheese and avocado. You can further lighten this choice by asking for no rice in your bowl.

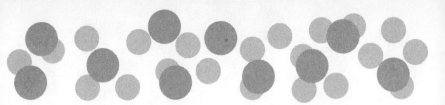

Mexican naked burrito (no rice)

Total calories = 320

Total fat = 12 g

Total carbs = 26 g

Total sugars = 8 g

MAKE IT YOURSELF SALAD

Naturally, a salad made with a balanced mix of lean protein, plenty of salad greens and controlled serves of fats from nuts, dressings, avocado and cheese can be a great lunch option. The key is to have a salad made to order and focus on a base mostly of low-calorie salad ingredients. Then add some lean protein such as eggs, tuna, turkey or chicken breast; some nutritious carbs from quinoa, sweet potato, corn or beans; and just one high-fat ingredient such as nuts, dressing, cheese or avocado. This mix will give you a lunch salad that contains fewer than 400 calories and a good amount of carbs and protein to help keep you full all afternoon.

Chicken, sweet potato and fetta salad

Total calories = 380

Total fat = 16 g

Total carbs =22 g

Total sugars = 2 g

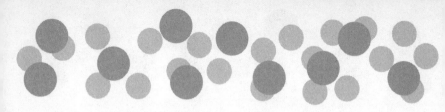

SUSHI

Sushi is one of the most popular default 'healthy' choices for a quick lunch on the run, but you do need to be careful as sushi rolls filled with fried fillings and tons of sticky white rice are not actually all that healthy. However, a serve of sashimi, along with some high protein edamame beans and a serve of seaweed salad is a high protein, high fibre, low-calorie lunch option that will keep you full for at least 2–3 hours.

Sashimi and Japanese salad

Total calories = 200–300

Total fat = 10 g

Total carbs = 15 g

Total sugars = 1 g

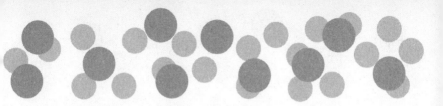

CHICKEN QUINOA SALAD

¼ cup quinoa, cooked

½ cucumber, sliced

1 tomato, chopped

80 g chicken breast, cooked and sliced

1 teaspoon raisins

1 tablespoon fresh parsley, chopped

1 tablespoon mint leaves

1 cup baby spinach leaves

2 tablespoons lemon juice

1 teaspoon extra virgin olive oil

1 Mix all ingredients together in bowl and dress with lemon juice and olive oil.

Serves 1

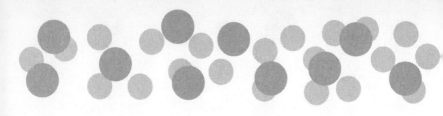

Halve your dinner

'Most of us eat so much during the day that we don't really need dinner.'

Halving the size of your dinner is a powerful weight-loss tool, but it doesn't have to be as dramatic as it seems. Simply reducing the size of your protein serve and aiming for a much larger serve of vegetables or salad is all you need to do, especially if you regularly find yourself eating late. Alternatively swap your dinner for soup a few nights a week to reduce your caloric intake while still enjoying a hearty meal.

Up to 30 per cent of lunch and dinner meals are eaten away from the home and restaurant meals have significantly more calories and fat than home-prepared options. To help counter this, aiming for a very light dinner the rest of the week is an easy way to strike a balance.

MAKING GOOD DINNER CHOICES			
REGULAR MEAL	**CALORIES**	**SMART SWAP**	**CALORIES**
Spaghetti bolognaise	400	3 meatballs and salad	200
Chicken schnitzel	420	100 g grilled chicken breast	190
Roast dinner	610	100 g grilled steak and salad	200
Pad thai	420	Thai beef salad	260

The best low-calorie dinners

GRILLED PRAWNS AND SALAD

While prawns have been considered taboo on many a low cholesterol diet, the truth is that prawns are an extremely nutrient-rich food that contains very few calories. With a large king prawn containing just 20–25 calories, you could easily enjoy a meal of 6–8 large prawns and salad and still consume just 200–250 calories. Or, a simple green prawn and vegetable stir-fry will again come in under 300 calories, which is particularly low for a dinner meal.

WHITE FISH AND VEGETABLES

Tuna and salmon are nutrient-rich types of fish, but their relatively high-fat content means they are also relatively high in calories. For example, a small serve of Atlantic salmon will contain at least 200 calories and 10–12 g of fat compared to a range of plain white fish fillets, which can contain half as many calories and almost no fat. Team your favourite grilled fish with steamed or stir-fried vegetables and you will have a filling, nutrient-rich meal for fewer than 300 calories per serve.

SOUP

It is not by chance that there are many, many diets that include soup as part of their regime. Broth and vegetable-based soups are exceptionally low in calories, rich in fibre and filling – with minimal calories. It appears that it is simply the volume of liquid consumed when we eat soup that helps to fill us up even though it has fewer calories than solid food. For

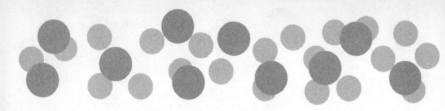

this reason, basing a couple of meals in your diet each week around soup is proven to enhance weight loss efforts.

ZUCCHINI NOODLE PASTA AND CAULIFLOWER RICE

For carb lovers, the thought of cutting back or completely eliminating carbohydrate-rich foods such as rice and pasta is enough to turn you off any diet. The good news is that you can swap rice and pasta for vegetable alternatives. For example, zucchini or pumpkin zoodles (now readily available in major supermarkets) or cauliflower rice are fibre-rich, low-calorie alternatives to carb-rich grains. Team your favourite rice or pasta vegetable alternative with a light, vegetable-rich sauce and voila, you have a low-calorie meal that will complement your weight loss attempts.

ROASTED VEGETABLE SALAD

Any meal that is based around vegetables will have fewer calories than a heavy rice or pasta meal. The key is to focus on the vegetables that have a particular high water content, such as beetroot, carrot, pumpkin, eggplant and literally any type of greens you can think of. If you simply roast your vegetables in a little olive oil and serve with a white cheese such as ricotta or cottage cheese, you will have another delicious, low-calorie meal.

WARM LAMB SALAD

150 g packet or 3 cups of assorted lettuce leaves

1 Lebanese cucumber, chopped

1 red capsicum, chopped

4 roma tomatoes, chopped

200 g pumpkin, roasted and diced

100 g low-fat fetta, chopped

400 g lean lamb fillets

1 tablespoon olive oil

tzatziki yoghurt dip, to serve

1 In a bowl, gently toss together the vegetables and fetta.

2 Finely slice the lamb fillets and brush all over with the oil. Sear lightly in a very hot wok or frying pan until medium-rare.

3 Arrange the lamb over the vegetables, drizzle with tzatziki and serve.

Serves 4

Know your quick and easy meals

'When you come home tired, you can order Thai, or throw a quick, nutritious meal together without excess calories.'

Life is busy and it's only likely to become more so. Less perceived time for food preparation tends to mean more takeaways, and more calories as a result. For this reason, knowing some quick and easy meals you can throw together in a few minutes is a crucial part of eating well for the larger part of the week.

When meals are prepared in a hurry, high-carb, low-vegetable options tend to fill our plates. Noodles, pasta or toast are easy favourites, but we need both a vegetable and a lean protein component if we are to keep the nutrition up and the calories down. Here are the best supermarket foods you can have at home for quick meals on the run.

OMELETTE

Eggs are one of nature's superfoods: packed full of key nutrients and protein. Grab an egg, whatever vegetables you have on hand that are easy to chop – like tomatoes, mushrooms, spinach or capsicum – and a little of your favourite cheese, and you have all the ingredients you need for a meal that can be made in 5 minutes and ticks a number of key nutritional boxes.

GRILL AND VEGETABLES

Whether you prefer lamb cutlets, lean sausages or a piece of chicken breast, any grilled lean meat when teamed with a basic salad or a packet or two of frozen vegetables is another nutritionally balanced meal that can be prepared in no time.

FROZEN FISH AND STIR-FRY

There is a wide range of plain frozen fish fillets, and when teamed with a stir-fry vegetable kit they make a tasty low-calorie meal. Alternatively, you can find fresh fish fillets or prawns in a light marinade in the fresh section of supermarkets. There are also frozen stir-fry vegetable kits that often come with a sauce to cook with.

NAKED BURGERS

There is a large range of lean beef and turkey burgers in supermakets these days, as well as pork and chicken meatballs, and any of these can make a healthy and delicious meal – minus the carb-rich bread rolls. Use lettuce, or even mushrooms, as your burger base. Teamed with plenty of salad, this is a protein-rich, tasty dinner that can be prepared in minutes.

MEXICAN FEAST

Forget slaving away over a pot of mince and vegetables for hours. Mix a few corn chips or taco shells, warm kidney beans, corn, chopped up vegetables, avocado, sour cream and a sprinkle of cheese for a meat-free meal, packed full of vegetable protein. It feels like a treat, but minus the calories and fat of takeaway Mexican.

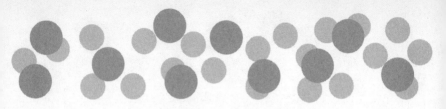

TASTY MINCE

2 teaspoons olive oil

1 onion, chopped

1 garlic clove, diced

500 g extra-lean mince

100 g salt-reduced tomato paste

200 g tin of diced tomatoes

2–3 cups mixed frozen vegetables

sprinkle of mozzarella and green salad to serve

1 Warm the oil in a frying pan. Add the onion and garlic and cook for 2 minutes. Add the mince and cook until browned.

2 Add the tomato paste, tomatoes and vegetables and simmer over a medium heat for 15–20 minutes, until cooked through.

3 Serve with a sprinkle of mozzarella and a large green salad.

Serves 4

PRAWNS AND ZUCCHINI

1 small zucchini, sliced

10 raw prawns, shelled and deveined

4–5 mushrooms, sliced

½ cup tomato pasta sauce

50 g low-fat fetta

Serves 1

1 Place a non-stick frying pan over a medium heat. Add the zucchini and sauté until just cooked through.

2 Add the prawns and cook, stirring, until they are translucent, for about 2–3 minutes.

3 Stir in the mushroom and pasta sauce and simmer until heated through, for about 3–5 minutes. Crumble the fetta over and serve.

ZUCCHINI OMELETTE

olive oil cooking spray

2 eggs, lightly beaten

½ small zucchini, finely grated

4 mushrooms, chopped

1 tomato, diced

1 red capsicum, diced

50 g low-fat ham, sliced

¼ cup low-fat grated cheese

Serves 1

1 Place a non-stick frying pan over a medium heat. Spray with cooking spray, then add the egg and swirl to coat the base of the pan.

2 Sprinkle the egg with the remaining ingredients. Cook for 2 minutes, or until the egg has set, then turn the omelette over and cook the other side.

3 Remove from the pan and set aside to cool slightly. Roll the omelette up, cut into slices and serve.

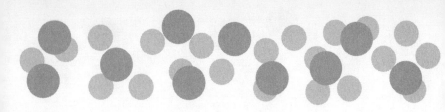

STUFFED POTATO

1 potato, with skin on, scrubbed well

100 g tin of tuna in oil, drained

1 small tomato, chopped

½ capsicum, chopped

¼ cup grated low-fat cheddar cheese,

Serves 1

1 Preheat the oven to 180ºC. Microwave the potato in its skin until tender, for about 5 minutes on medium.

2 Slice the potato open and fill with the tuna, tomato and capsicum. Sprinkle with the cheese.

3 Bake for 5–10 minutes, or until the cheese has melted.

Soup it up

'Who would have thought that a humble bowl of soup could offer so many weight-loss benefits?'

A dietitian always has tricks in her or his toolbox. My favourite is a recipe that can relatively quickly shift fluid, leaving you feeling lighter and in a good place psychologically to continue with your weight loss regime.

Vegetable-based soups have an extremely high nutrient content, are very low in calories and provide bulk to prevent you feeling hungry and deprived as you would using meal-replacement shakes. Studies show that enjoying a broth-based soup before a meal can reduce caloric intake for the remainder of the meal by 20 per cent. As favoured by the skinny French, soups that have a base of leeks, onions and/or celery (see recipe on page 106) are particularly high in the mineral potassium. Potassium helps rid the body of the excess fluid many of us carry thanks to a high-salt diet and lack of activity, but dropping as little as 500 g, even if it is just fluid, can make us feel lighter and leaner instantly.

For those wanting a more intense regime or short-term results, vegetable soup can replace two meals a day for 5–7 days without negative side effects.

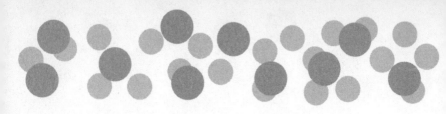

CHICKEN AND VEGETABLE SOUP

2 skinless chicken breast fillets, diced

4 cups (1 litre) reduced-salt chicken stock

1 tablespoon canola oil

2 leeks, white part only, finely sliced

2 carrots, diced

2 celery stalks, diced

3 garlic cloves, crushed

6 cups or 200 g young green salad leaves, such as watercress, rocket, sorrel and baby spinach, finely chopped

3 tablespoons fresh pesto

Serves 6

1 Place the chicken in a saucepan and pour in just enough stock to cover. Poach gently for 10 minutes, or until the chicken is just cooked. Set aside to cool.

2 Heat the oil in a large saucepan. Add the leek and gently sauté until soft, for about 2 minutes. Stir in the carrot, celery and garlic.

3 Strain the chicken poaching stock through a fine sieve, then add to the vegetables with the remaining stock. Simmer for 10 minutes. Stir in the greens and simmer for a further 10 minutes.

4 Shred the chicken and add it to the soup. Stir in the pesto and season to taste with plenty of freshly ground black pepper.

Learn to love salads

'Want to slash your calories at dinner?
Just add a salad – it's that simple.'

If you consider that simply eating a large green salad before you tuck into
your dinner can reduce your total energy intake by as much as 120 calories,
it may be worth chopping up a few extra greens each week. The humble
lettuce not only adds bulk to your diet and helps you to eat less, but it
is extremely low in calories. Adding extra salad to both your lunch and
evening meal will improve the nutritional profile of your diet in general.

MAKING THE PERFECT SALAD MEAL

Step 1 – Salad greens Whether you choose cos lettuce, rocket or English
spinach, follow this mantra: the darker the leaves, the better they are for
you. Salad leaves are rich sources of fibre, vitamins C and K and generally
form the base of a salad that will help to keep you full for a number of
hours after eating it.

Step 2 – Plenty of brightly coloured vegetables The more you include,
the better the salad will be for you – carrots, cucumber, celery, tomatoes,
beetroot, pumpkin and capsicum. If you find yourself throwing out too
much fresh produce, try making one large salad base each week and
adding the wetter items, such as tomatoes, later. This way you always have

some salad ready to go and can even add it to sandwiches, wraps and crackers as extra fillers throughout the day.

Step 3 – Carbs for energy A plain salad enjoyed at lunch without any bread, crackers or other forms of carbohydrate may appear to be the most healthy, calorie-controlled option but remember that not eating adequate carbs throughout the day can leave you feeling unsatisfied and more likely to binge later in the afternoon. Adding a small amount of low-GI carbohydrate to your salad in the form of sweet potato, corn or beans, or enjoying your salad with a slice of wholegrain bread or crackers will complete your meal perfectly.

Step 4 – Lean protein for nutrition A small tin of tuna or salmon, 1–2 eggs or a palm-sized serve of lean meat or chicken are not only a filling component of your salad but also have much to offer nutritionally. Protein foods are rich sources of iron, zinc, vitamin B12 and omega-3 fats. Remember, the less processed the better, and if you choose tuna in olive oil, make sure that you drain off the extra oil to avoid a fat overload.

Step 5 – Added fats Salad dressings, nuts and cheese may all be tasty additions to your salad but they are high-fat choices and can quickly turn your healthy salad into a calorie overload if you're not careful. Aim for just one of these additions to your salad and remember that olive oil and walnuts are the two best high-fat additions due to their optimal fat profile.

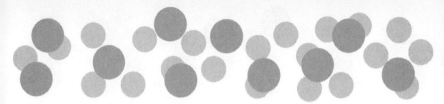

AND THE ONES TO AVOID …

Chicken Caesar Salad This remains one of the most popular salad choices on the menu, but you do not need a science degree to figure out that a mix of creamy dressing, bacon, cheese, toasted bread and oil may not always be the healthiest option. With just half a cup of Caesar salad equating to as much as 13 g of fat, an average serve of Caesar salad can give you up to 40–50 g of fat with relatively small amounts of protein and fibre.

Pasta salad The name kind of gives it away – despite being described as a 'salad', nutritionally it lacks the fibre and vegetable bulk to consider it a light lunch choice. Pasta salad is a high-carbohydrate, low-protein lunch option that can contain as much as 20 g of fat and 30 g of total carbohydrates (2–3 slices of bread) in a single cup. With it commonly being dressed with high-fat ingredients including pesto, mayonnaise or other creamy dressings, and including very few vegetables, you are best to leave pasta to a great Italian meal and focus your 'salad' elsewhere.

Spinach, pumpkin and fetta salad This one is a little misleading because all the green makes it look like an exceptionally healthy choice, but the addition of nuts, dressing, cheese and avocado makes this salad a high-fat meal with little protein or salad bulk to keep you full. When it comes to added fats, whether it is avocado, dressing, nuts or cheese, each will contain 5–10 g of fat per serve. This salad could be giving you as much as

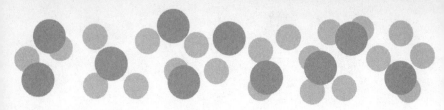

40–50 g of fat in a single serve – close to your entire daily requirement. See recipe opposite for a tasty alternative that will help you keep things light.

Cous cous, quinoa or brown rice salad Grains including brown rice, quinoa or cous cous offer much nutritionally, but they are carbohydrate-rich foods: meaning they are concentrated, fuel-rich foods. For example, just half a cup of any of these grains has equivalent carbohydrates to two slices of bread. The issue with salads that are based on these grains is that they tend to be heavy in carbs and low in protein and vegetables. The average brown rice or quinoa salad contains 50 g or more of carbs, or the equivalent of four or more slices of bread. If weight control is your goal and you spend much of the day sitting, leave your carbs as a side and base your salads around vegetables and lean proteins.

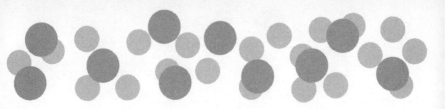

HALOUMI, PUMPKIN, SWEET POTATO AND CHICKEN SALAD

1 small sweet potato (200 g), peeled and cut into 2–3 cm cubes

600 g pumpkin, cut into 2–3 cm cubes

olive oil spray

⅔ cup reduced fat Greek yoghurt

3 tablespoons lemon juice, to taste

2 teaspoons crushed garlic, to taste

350 g chicken breast fillet, cut into thin strips

150 g haloumi, sliced

4 cups rocket and baby spinach leaves

¼ cup pine nuts, lightly toasted

Serves 4

1 Lightly spray sweet potato and pumpkin cubes with oil and bake in a pre-heated, fan-forced oven at 200°C, for 50–60 minutes, or until cooked through. Set aside.

2 To prepare the dressing, mix together the yoghurt, 1 tablespoon lemon juice and 1 teaspoon garlic.

3 In a bowl, marinate the chicken strips in 2 tablespoons lemon juice and 1 teaspoon garlic.

4 Lightly spray a non-stick fry pan with oil and place over medium heat. Cook sliced haloumi for 1 minute on each side or until golden. Set aside and cover with foil to keep warm.

5 Using the same pan, cook the marinated chicken strips.

6 Gently toss together the mixed leaves, pumpkin and toasted pine nuts. Divide evenly into four portions. Top with a portion of haloumi, chicken and a few dollops of yoghurt dressing.

Embrace a sugar detox

'If you constantly crave sweet foods, it may be time to do a sugar detox.'

You know the drill: you start the day with a caramel latte, are hanging out for some banana bread at morning tea and feel like you are going to die at 3 or 4 pm if you don't get your hands on some diet soft drink and a chocolate bar. If this sounds even remotely familiar, you may need a sugar detox to take control of your tastebuds and eating habits.

From the time we are given our first taste of mashed banana or custard as babies we are embracing a reward system that programs us to seek pleasure from sweet foods. It doesn't matter if you get your sweet fix from diet yoghurt, fruit, low-fat banana bread, low-calorie biscuits or low-fat dessert, the fact that you are constantly searching for sweet taste sensations is the real issue. Until you alter this drive, you are going to be constantly craving and seeking out more and more sweet foods to satisfy the desire.

Generally it will take at least 2–3 days without any sweet food for you to no longer be searching for it. This means you're going to have to work through a mini-detox and possibly some withdrawal symptoms, including headaches, cravings, irritability and fluctuating blood sugar levels. As you submit to this process, keep in mind that the need for sweet foods can be

SUGARS IN FOOD		
FOOD	CALORIES	TEASPOONS OF SUGAR
200 ml low-fat fruit yoghurt	170	5
1 cup Nutrigrain cereal	110	2
Glass of cordial	100	5
2 plain biscuits	80	3
2 Weight Watchers biscuits	36	2
2 jelly snakes	40	2
1 tbsp tomato sauce	20	1

shifted by tasting savoury and salty foods, anything that shifts the palate. Useful foods at this time include those with strong mint flavours, green tea or savoury proteins.

The good news is that once you've detoxed from sweet foods, over time you'll notice that you get the same amount of pleasure from naturally sweet foods like yoghurt and fruit as you once did from cakes and biscuits. You will also need far less of the very sweet foods to get the same hit you once needed. Ultimately this means less high-calorie sweet food will be entering your mouth, which ultimately means less weight long-term and a new you who is no longer controlled by your sugar cravings.

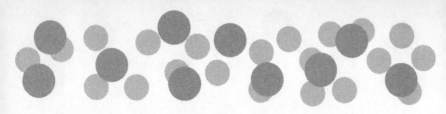

THE SUGAR SWAP	
Fruit muesli	Plain oats
Fruit yoghurt	Natural yoghurt
Sugar	Cinnamon or vanilla
Milk chocolate	70% dark chocolate
Dried fruit	Fresh fruit
Muesli bars	Nut-based snack bars
Rice crackers	Roasted chickpeas
Wraps	Rye crackers
Mayonnaise	Avocado
Sweet chilli sauce	Chilli sauce

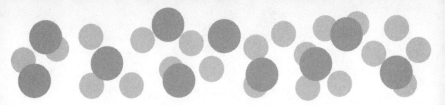

Are you having any extras?

'All the hidden extras really do add up.'

A spread of margarine here, a dollop of sauce there and before you know it you have an extra 200 calories a day, which is the difference between weight loss and not. There is no denying that these little extras make our food taste better, but as these small additions gradually become larger, they really add up.

Let's start with spreads. Butter or margarine contains at least 30 calories per teaspoon. Unless you are being mindful you are likely to be using far more than you think and in many cases just adding calories rather than flavour. High-calorie spreads including nut pastes, jam, honey and chocolate spreads are all recipes for disaster when it comes to extra calories. Such options offer little nutritionally, and they are extras we can easily do without once we are basing our food choices around a good carb and protein balance.

Sugar in tea and coffee is another trap to avoid. What should be a level 5 g teaspoon is more likely to be heaped and the more you have, the more you want. Swap to sugar cubes or wean off altogether.

Avocado is another addition we take for granted. The ideal 20 g serve is more likely to become half the fruit added to salads and sandwiches rather than the thin spread or light scattering it should be.

Sauces are the next issue. Soy, oyster, tomato, barbecue – you are adding about 10–20 calories per teaspoon. Start to measure your portions so you know how much you are really using.

Olive oil can quickly add up too. While celebrity chefs heartily pour litres of the stuff into their cooking, if you consider that just 1 teaspoon of oil contains more than 40 calories, you can see how easy it is to go overboard. Use spray oils where possible and measure your quantities when adding oil to pastas or salad.

EXTRAS CALORIE COUNTER		
EXTRA	CALORIES	FAT (g)
1 tbsp peanut butter	155	13
¼ avocado	130	14
1 tbsp jam	70	0
1 syrup shot in coffee	65	0
1 tsp olive oil	40	4
1 tsp margarine	35	4
1 tbsp sweet chilli sauce	25	<1
1 tbsp tomato sauce	20	0
1 tsp sugar	17	0

Go smaller

'We eat far more than we think we do.'

Serving sizes have become a whole lot bigger. Soft drinks now come in 600 ml bottles as the norm, potato chips in 100 g packets and even the average slice of bread won't fit in a regular toaster. Yet while servings are increasing, we are moving less so actually need fewer calories to fuel our muscles. It's not difficult to see how weight gain is almost inevitable.

Behavioural research has repeatedly shown that people will eat what is in front of them. For example, if you have chocolates on your desk in a glass container instead of a ceramic container, you will eat double the number simply because you can see them. You are not weak, you are just human.

A realistic weight-loss trick that allows you to enjoy your favourite foods while controlling your weight is to simply monitor your portion sizes, at every meal, every day. Reducing caloric intake gradually over time and maintaining the reduction is ultimately the trick to long-term weight control.

So how can you get a firm grasp of your own portion distortion? Let's start with breakfast. Measure just ¾ cup of breakfast cereal and serve it in a small shallow bowl, rather than a soup-style bowl. Choosing smaller slices of bread and smearing no more than a teaspoon of butter on your

toast means you will have saved yourself more than 50 calories. That may not seem like much but if you save this amount of energy every day, that is more than 250 calories per week, or almost 2 kg of body weight over the course of a year.

Next is your choice of coffee cup size. Large coffees contain as many calories as a meal, yet few of us count them as such. Generally coffee shops will offer regular-sized cups that contain at least 250 calories more than small cups. Always ask for small coffees.

Then onto morning tea. Large packets of potato chips, biscuits, cheese, nuts and lollies are setting you up to fail. Individual-sized portions of yoghurt, cheese and crackers are convenient ways to make sure you do not over-serve yourself. If you are craving something sweet, remember that the most pleasure is derived from your first few mouthfuls of food so just a third or half a slice of cake should be more than enough to satisfy any cravings.

At lunchtime remember that sandwiches purchased from sandwich bars provide double the amount of calories you really need from your lunch, so you may only need to eat half a large sandwich with a piece of fruit to satisfy you. If you are making your lunch, a few crackers or a slice of flat bread is often all you need to keep you full for another 2–3 hours. Other high risk foods that tend to be overeaten during the day include nuts (10 is a serve), avocado (¼ is a serve) and salad dressings (you only need a teaspoon).

For your evening meal, try weighing your portions of meat to grasp how much you are actually having. Women will need just 100–150 g and men 150–200 g of lean meat, chicken or fish. Serves of Atlantic salmon and steak can often be double this size.

Finally your treats at night – tubs of ice-cream and blocks of chocolate are asking for trouble. If you do enjoy a sweet treat at night, always look for portion-controlled servings and stick to less than 100 calories.

SIMPLE CHANGES, HUGE CALORIE REDUCTION

The table below is a reminder of how some simple changes can have a massive impact on calorie intake over the course of a year. These figures are based on estimates of consumption frequency over a week.

CALORIE SAVING SWAPS			
SWAP	FOR	CALORIES SAVED	BODY FAT EQUIV. /YEAR
1 tbsp oil	1 tsp oil	125	2 kg
200 g meat	150 g meat	75	1.8 kg
1 large slice bread	1 small slice bread	40	1.2 kg
Margarine on toast	Olive oil spread on toast	35	2 kg
1 cup cereal	¾ cup cereal	25	0.25 kg
Tea with milk	Herbal tea	10	0.6 kg
1 heaped tsp sugar	1 cube sugar	5	1.6 kg

BEEF AND SNOW PEA STIR-FRY

500 g lean rump steak

1 tablespoon brown sugar

2 tablespoons sunflower or rice bran oil

250 g snow peas

2 large carrots, thinly sliced on the diagonal

2 red capsicums, cut into chunks

⅓ (80 ml) oyster sauce

2 tablespoons soy sauce

½ cup steamed brown rice to serve

1 Rub the beef all over with the sugar and half the oil and cut into thin strips.

2 Heat a wok and lightly stir-fry the beef and transfer to a plate.

3 Heat the remaining oil in the wok. Quickly stir-fry the vegetables in the oyster sauce and soy sauce until just tender.

4 Return the beef to the wok. Toss until well combined and heated through. Serve immediately, with steamed brown rice.

Serves 4

Quality over quantity

'If you always go for quality over quantity you won't go wrong.'

Despite what we are often told, there are actually no 'bad' foods – there are foods that supply the body with more calories than others, and there are foods that supply the body with more nutrients than others; but at the end of the day, there is not one food that makes you fat or that should never be eaten. Having said that, there are styles of eating that are closely linked to consuming too many calories on a regular basis. These are what ultimately result in unwanted weight gain.

A common scenario that presents with overweight clients is that they find themselves eating foods because the food is what they think they 'should' be eating, as opposed to what they 'feel' like eating. Then, as their actual craving has not been fulfilled, they end up eating an extra sweet treat in addition to their meal or snack. This results in too much food in total and weight gain over time. Individuals who appear to eat what they like, when they like, often avoid the overeating that occurs when you do not listen to your natural appetite signals.

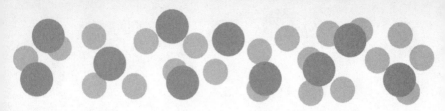

This approach does not mean that you should be binge eating a block of chocolate every time you crave some, but it does mean that if you feel like some chocolate, you should have it. The key to avoiding overeating is to choose good quality chocolate, in portion-controlled quantities, and to sit and enjoy it properly.

Once you accept that there are no foods you cannot eat, ask yourself what you really feel like eating when you do get hungry and really consider which food choice will satisfy you. This is when you will have finally reached a state of self control with your eating. Remember, food is meant to nourish the body and be enjoyed; it is as simple as that.

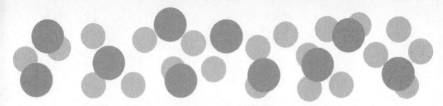

Change your food thinking

1   Stop thinking of food as 'good' and 'bad': instead consider 'everyday' foods and 'sometimes' foods.

2   Differentiate regular, daily eating occasions from special occasions where you may indulge.

3   If you overdo it, have a day of eating just light soups or salad.

4   Include a small treat in your daily eating plan such as a few pieces of chocolate or glass of wine.

5   Practise keeping high-fat treats in the house and not eating them just because they are there. This helps normalise these foods rather than viewing them as 'treats' that should not be eaten.

6   Stop hiding food; you know it is there.

7   If you crave sweet foods, satisfy the food craving but also make it part of a balanced snack so you are kept full for a couple of hours after eating it.

8   Always ask yourself, 'What do I really feel like eating?'

9   If you are experiencing constant cravings, check if your baseline diet is well balanced – an unbalanced diet can result in constant hunger and food cravings.

10 Remember the mantra of 'quality over quantity' when indulging – if it is not great quality chocolate, cakes, cheese or desserts, don't waste your calories. Save them for something you love to eat.

Get your timing right

'Ideally we need 10–12 hours without food overnight.'

Long gone are the days when we ate breakfast at 7 am, lunch at midday and dinner by 6 pm. Nowadays breakfast is more likely to be enjoyed with coffee at 9 am, lunch by 2 pm or even 3 pm as the demands of the day see time getting away from us, and dinner by 8, if we are lucky. Long commutes and frantic lives mean that we eat far more sporadically than we used to, which has much more of a negative impact on our weight than we may realise.

The human body is regulated according to a circadian rhythm – this means that our basic physiological processes, including our hormones, are controlled according to a 24-hour body clock. We are programmed to burn more fuel in the first half of the day, and to store it later. It means the body is also programmed to have periods of time without food (overnight) and that there are times the body is in store and repair mode as opposed to mobilise fuel and burn it mode. Nothing we do significantly changes this. We may do shift work and eat throughout the night, but the body will remain programmed to not be burning as much energy overnight (and more likely to store food consumed at this time).

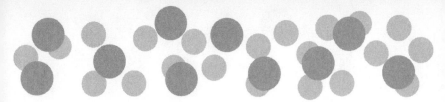

It is for this reason that modern life and the random, if not constant, feeding that we expose the body to, is conducive to weight gain over time. Often we eat far more food late in the day than we do the morning; we do not give the body the long periods of time it needs overnight without food to allow the hormones that control fat metabolism to return to baseline levels. Focusing on eating the right things at the right times of day is one of the most powerful things you can do to control your weight long-term.

EAT EARLY

To tap into your natural metabolism, the best thing you can do is eat something early in the day – 9 am or 10 am is too late for breakfast. Ideally, we need to eat by 7 am or 8 am to get our system going each morning. One of the reasons you feel hungrier on days when you eat breakfast early is that your metabolism has been given a boost.

PRIORITISE LUNCH

If you start the day early, forget eating your lunch at 2 pm or 3 pm – it is too late. Generally speaking, you will feel hungry 3–4 hours after your first meal, which means that most of us will benefit from an early lunch. Another option for particularly early risers is to enjoy two small lunches: one at 11–12 pm and one at 2–3 pm – this also helps avoid unnecessary snacking throughout the day.

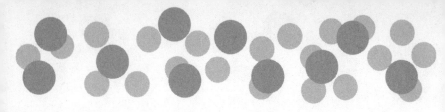

KEEP AN EYE ON DINNER

Ideally the body needs at least 10–12 hours without any food overnight, which for most of us means we need to eat our dinner by 8 pm, but the earlier the better. If you routinely find yourself eating dinner after 8 pm, another option is to make lunch your main meal of the day and then enjoy a lighter meal such as soup, an omelette or salad later in the evening. Similarly, for those working a long day, enjoying a substantial snack at 3–4 pm, followed by a light dinner later, will help give your body the time overnight it needs to support weight control (as opposed to the gradual weight gain that we see with heavy meals consumed late at night).

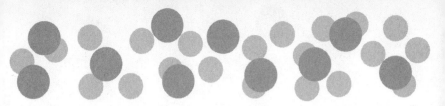

Are the people in your life making you fat?

'We become like the people we spend our time with.'

A couple of years ago a long-term study published in *The New England Journal of Medicine* found a powerful link between an individual's weight and the weight of those closest to them. When researchers involved in the Framingham Heart Study, which has followed more than 15,000 Framingham residents since 1948, took a closer look at the data, tracking the social connections of participants who gained or lost weight, it became clear that individuals did not become obese randomly. Rather, groups of people would become obese together or even lose weight together. The study showed that when a Framingham resident became obese, his or her friends were 57 per cent more likely to become obese too.

These findings tell us one thing – that we become like the people we spend our time with. And as such, there is a wide range of influencers who may be playing a bigger role in your health and your weight than you may have previously been aware of.

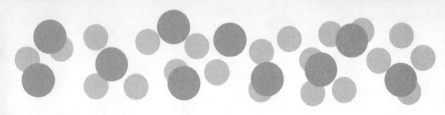

YOUR FRIENDS

Put most simply, if your friends regularly exercise and make healthy meal choices when eating out, you are far more likely to keep your weight under control than if your friends make poor food choices, don't move much and carry extra weight. Friends can also – consciously or unconsciously – play a 'feeder' role in which they encourage you to eat foods you may not really want to. For this reason, it is important to be honest and transparent with those closest to us. Be confident to stand up and say that you are keen to stick to your diet. Look for active social engagements if you are keen to lose or control your weight.

YOUR KIDS

As parents we are often guilty of forgetting to take care of ourselves: if we are not careful, our diet can quickly become a mix of kids' foods, sugary drinks and treats. Child-friendly restaurants and easy takeaways tend to offer high-carb, high-fat foods that we end up eating too, by default. The easiest way to avoid snacking on meals for kids is to ensure your nutritional needs are satisfied first. While it may go against the grain to do so, choosing your cuisine first, packing your own snacks and eating your breakfast before the kids are the easiest ways to avoid eating highly processed kids' foods too frequently. Mind you, ideally the kids will not be eating too much of these things either!

YOUR PARTNER

Partners are notorious for playing a lead role in sabotaging each other's diets, especially when they do not want to make healthy choices themselves. You need to be strong here – prepare separate meals if you have to. And be honest: point out to them that bringing chocolates and treats home, or tempting you with alcohol when you are trying to have an alcohol-free night, is not helpful and, actually, quite selfish.

YOUR COLLEAGUES

The fact that so many of us spend so many hours each week at work can be a disaster when it comes to our diets if our workplaces are not all that healthy. The combination of fundraising chocolates, regular birthday cakes, vending machines and office feeders can be a disaster when it comes to our overall calorie intake. Avoid overeating at the office by planning ahead, taking your food where you can and saying no to the incessant bakers.

YOUR FAMILY

The powerful programming effects of our early experiences with food can mean that we instantly return to childhood food habits when we are in the presence of family. Then there are also the relatives who routinely

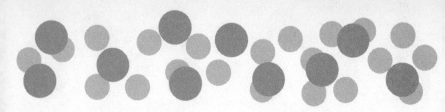

offer you large volumes of delicious home-cooked, heavy foods that are impossible to refuse. When possible say no, especially to empty-calorie foods such as snacks, lollies and chocolates. When you can't, focus on portion control and bulking up your plate with extra vegetables and salad.

LOW-CALORIE DINNER OMELETTE

olive oil cooking spray

1 egg, lightly beaten with
a dash of low-fat milk

½ small zucchini, grated

1 tomato, chopped

¼ red capsicum, chopped

2 tablespoons grated
low-fat cheddar cheese

Serves 1

1 Place a non-stick frying pan over a medium heat. Coat pan with cooking spray, then add the egg and swirl to coat the base of the pan.

2 Sprinkle the egg with the zucchini, tomato, capsicum and cheese. Cook for 2 minutes, or until the egg has set, then turn the omelette over and cook the other side. Serve with a salad.

Be smart when eating out

'For those who eat out regularly, knowing what to order goes a long way to keeping your weight under control.'

We all need to know some simple tricks to master the delicate balance of enjoying our favourite cuisines and restaurants without a complete calorie overload. Unfortunately restaurant meals often mean extra calories thanks to larger portion sizes, the liberal use of oil, butter and sauces as well as numerous courses.

CHOOSE YOUR CUISINES CAREFULLY

While we are blessed with a myriad of options when it comes to eating out, some cuisines offer better choices than others. Indian, Chinese and Thai food in particular tend to be extremely high in fat, due to the use of coconut milk and batters, as well as the large volumes of oil used. When high-fat curries and fried foods are eaten with large amounts of white rice, noodles and bread, it's easy to see how an energy overload can result. Ideally such high-fat cuisines need to be consumed sparingly – just once or twice a month. Be mindful of avoiding the fried choices on the menu. Instead look for plain vegetable curries and stir-fries and try enjoying them with just a small scoop of either rice, noodles or bread.

LOOK FOR THE LIGHT OPTIONS

Lighter options that can be enjoyed more regularly include Japanese and Greek cuisines, as these tend to have a much wider range of menu items that will allow you to make healthier choices. Any sort of raw fish, grilled meat or seafood will be a great choice, especially when teamed with a large portion of vegetables or salad. If you are trying to lose weight, be direct with friends and colleagues when choosing places to dine. Encourage them to visit a restaurant you know has healthy options.

SIZE IS EVERYTHING

One of the biggest issues with eating out is that we tend to eat much more. Few of us really need both an entrée as well as a main course and for most of us an entrée-sized portion of heavier foods such as pasta or risotto will be more than sufficient. If the serves of pasta, rice or meat are far larger than you need, before you start your meal, visualise how much of the portion you will eat, and then take the excess off your plate and share with your fellow diners. Otherwise learn to be comfortable leaving some food on your plate if you know you are not hungry enough to eat it. If you must have an entrée, look for lighter options such as a few grilled seafood pieces, a soup or salad. When it comes to dessert, remember that the most pleasure is gained in the first few mouthfuls, so if you really spot something you love on the menu, share with as many people as possible.

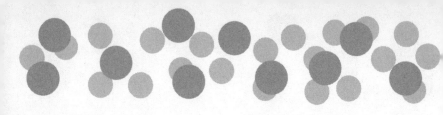

VEGETABLES, VEGETABLES, VEGETABLES

One of the biggest issues with meals consumed away from the home is that they rarely contain the amounts of vegetables or salad we need for good health and to help us feel full. Even though they can be expensive when ordered as sides, it's worth ordering extras to help bulk up your meal so you're not tempted by chips or bread. When eating heavier cuisines such as Indian and Thai, always order an extra vegetable-based dish to reduce the amount of heavy curry and rice that you are likely to eat.

PLAN AHEAD

If you really struggle to limit yourself when you are out, another powerful psychological technique is to plan in advance what will be the best choice for you prior to arriving at the restaurant. This way you won't be overwhelmed with options and make a rash decision. Also when you

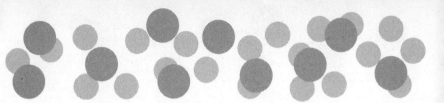

arrive remember how dreadful you feel when you overeat – this can be a strong deterrent.

WHAT'S THE OCCASION?

Perhaps the most important thing to consider when you're dining out is whether it's a special occasion, or just a regular occurrence. For special occasions enjoyed at amazing restaurants, look for ways to make your meal well-balanced and avoid overeating, but of course take the opportunity to enjoy dessert and other treats you would not usually have. It's the weekly Thai or trip to the local restaurant that does more damage than the one-off celebrations.

Top tips for eating out

1   Never go to a restaurant starving. Have a small snack 1–2 hours before to take the edge off your hunger.

2   Be direct with friends when they're making restaurant choices – remember that both Indian and Thai foods are exceptionally high in fat.

3   If you love eating bread, try doing what the Italians do – take the middle out and just enjoy the crust.

4   Order as much extra salad and as many vegetables as you can to bulk up your plate.

5   Aim to be the last to finish your meal, eating slowly, placing your knife and fork down between each mouthful and chewing everything well.

6   Be mindful that restaurant food is often very salty, so drink at least three glasses of water throughout the meal to help flush away the salt and avoid bloating.

7   If you have overdone things, just make sure your next meal is a light soup or salad to help compensate for the extra calories.

8   Sit with the person who eats the least and likes to eat healthily. You are likely to be influenced by what those around you are ordering so this will help keep you on track.

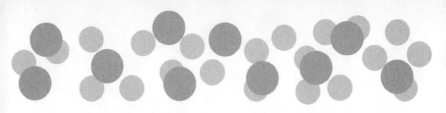

ENERGY AND FAT CONTENT OF COMMON MEALS OUT			
COMMON CHOICE	BETTER CHOICE	CALORIE SAVING	FAT SAVING (g)
Pad thai	Chicken stir-fry	350	8
Chicken teriyaki	8-pack sushi	300	17
Butter chicken	Tandoori chicken	200	17
Pesto pasta	Spaghetti bolognaise	250	24
3-piece KFC feed	4-piece Oporto pack	600	49
4 slices Meat Lovers pizza	Chicken kebab	400	29
Thai green curry	Pork stir-fry in soy sauce	0	35

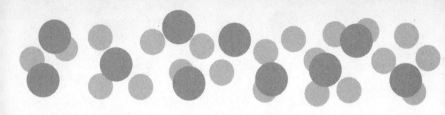

Take a meal off

'Restriction rarely works long-term – we need to manage our diet sustainably to control our weight for good.'

Often when we begin a weight-loss program, we expect to feel deprived, to not be able to eat any of our favourite foods and that the diet will be completely ruined if we eat something that is not on the list. But the truth is that the body actually doesn't respond well to long periods of strict calorie restriction.

Research shows that long periods of time with too few calories can result in the brain releasing neurotransmitters that make you want to eat. It appears that when the body thinks it is starving, it is powerfully driven to seek food, which may be the reason dieters face the intense hunger that makes it so challenging to stay on track after experiencing initial weight loss.

A very easy way to overcome this physiological signalling is to include a meal in your regular diet plan that is 'free', or has more calories than you have been limiting yourself to for the other 6 days of the week. Not only does this give you the freedom to enjoy a meal out or special celebration, but it also gives your body the message that it is not starving and should burn up energy and extra fat as usual – a win–win situation.

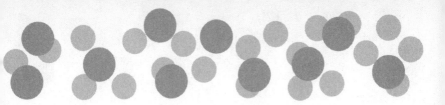

Now, please note that the suggestion is to have one meal off – not a whole day, not a four-course buffet, just one meal. This may mean including some carbohydrates at night, it may mean adding in a slice of birthday cake or including a couple of alcoholic drinks on a night out. Overall you should aim for no more than 200–250 extra calories. Follow this meal with some extra movement and then get straight back on to your program. Such a change will not negatively affect your weight-loss attempt, in fact it may even enhance it.

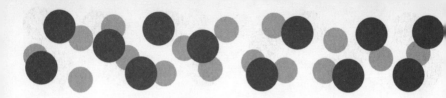

your
BEHAVIOUR

'Only you have control over
what goes into your mouth.'

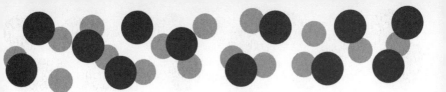

CHECK YOURSELF

How many times a day does
food enter your mouth? 142

Know your eating style 143

Food habits that make you fat 147

Are your hormones making
you fat? 151

SUSTAINABLE CHANGE

Reset your hunger switch 154

Consider a fast 157

Mindless munching 160

Develop your self-regulation
skills 163

Build your willpower 165

Managing cravings 169

Learn to stop overeating 171

Think thin 174

Expect a plateau 178

How many times a day does food enter your mouth?

'Once you count the snacks, treats, meals and drinks – many of us are eating 20–30 times a day.'

For one day I want you to keep a record of the number of times any sort of food enters your mouth. Not just your meals, but all the coffees and tea with milk or sugar, snacks, leftovers and treats that slip in over the day. Many of my clients were astounded to find after keeping this record that food was entering their mouths as many as 20–30 times each day, when the number should be more like 6–7 times at most.

The body is programmed to eat a meal and then nothing for at least 2–3 hours. Constant nibbling between meals and snacks disrupts the natural digestive process. When we eat, insulin is secreted to take glucose to the muscles. Insulin is a fat-storing hormone, so every time you eat something, no matter how small, insulin will be secreted, and the more insulin, the more fat storage that occurs over time.

Aim to eat only every 2–3 hours with nothing except water or herbal tea in between. This will allow your digestive hormones to function efficiently and help you experience your natural hunger and satiety signals – the best guides when it comes to when and how much you should eat.

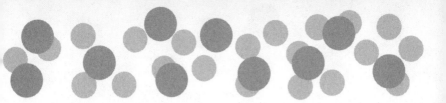

Know your eating style

'Some of us binge, others restrict, others need to try everything. Identifying your eating pattern will help you get your weight under control for good.'

Everyone has a different eating style depending on food preferences, what we're taught as children and who we spend our time with, but does your eating style prevent weight loss? Once your pattern has been identified, you can generally manage it with a few basic behavioural strategies.

RESTRICTED EATING

Restrictive eaters base their food choices on what they think they should eat as opposed to what they feel like eating. They tend to have strict food rules but can be prone to overeating when one of these rules is broken. Restrictive eaters are often on a diet, may avoid social situations for fear of not having access to the food they think they should be eating and spend far too much time calculating the fat and calorie content of their diets.

A good starting point is to ask yourself, 'What do I really feel like eating?' Try to remove the cognitive programming entrenched in your mind that tells you certain foods are bad. Once you start challenging these beliefs and eating foods you normally avoid, you will not feel out of control if you do try a dessert or eat a controlled portion of carbohydrates at dinner. Always remember that there are no strict rules about what we should and

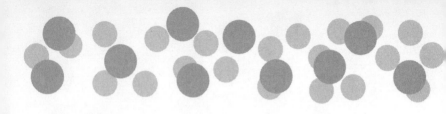

shouldn't eat – there are balanced meals with everyday foods, and other foods that we eat sometimes in controlled amounts.

EMOTIONAL EATING

Some of us eat less when we are sad, stressed or lonely while some of us eat more. Emotional eating is frequently reported as a behavioural side effect of emotional distress, and if not identified and managed early can result in extra body weight courtesy of chocolates, ice-creams and biscuits – the most common foods sought out by emotional eaters.

The first thing to do is identify the emotional triggers that lead you to eat high-calorie food. Then you can practise having a 'time out' in between the trigger and the eating – try calling a friend, getting out of the house or office (a change in environment works very effectively) or writing down the pros and cons of eating your desired treat. This breathing space makes it much easier to think rationally about eating rather than rushing to the fridge and downing a tub of ice-cream. If you are prone to emotional overeating, never keep your comfort foods in the house. Having to go out to buy them puts time in between the crisis point and when the food is available, which will help you to make a rational decision not to binge.

THE SERIAL DIETER

You name it, the serial dieter has tried it! Low-carb, high-protein, cabbage only – but the serial dieter never seems to lose weight. Too much energy is spent on fad diets instead of developing long-term healthy eating behaviour.

If you are a serial dieter, think about all the precious time and energy (not to mention money) you have wasted on these programs for no outcome. In fact, serial dieting tends to have a negative impact on metabolic rate long-term and can be particularly limiting psychologically if each diet has resulted in failure. If you are serious about getting healthy, book yourself into a dietitian and get a balanced, personalised food plan to deal with your weight issues once and for all.

THE EVENING BINGER

Evening bingers eat next to nothing all day, arrive home famished and eat everything in sight. Consuming a disproportionate number of calories during the second half of the day means low energy levels in the morning and long-term weight gain, as high-calorie foods are often chosen at this time, when your body has switched from fat burning to fat storage mode.

If you are a night binger, you need to get organised and support your metabolism rather than sabotage it. Practise planning ahead each day so you have all the food supplies you need for at least three meals each day. Try having a protein-rich snack such as a nut bar, milk-based drink or protein bar on the way home from work so you don't walk in the door ravenous. Like emotional eaters, you may find it helps to not keep easy-to-eat snacks such as biscuits, dips, chocolates and potato chips at home as they are too easy to overeat when you're starving.

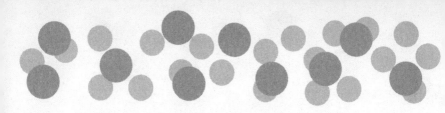

THE HEALTH FANATIC

Health fanatics may look fabulous from a distance but a closer look can reveal dry skin, fatigue and low moods as the obsession with all things natural and healthy has resulted in a life without much pleasure. While eating nutritionally balanced food should be a goal for all of us, taking it to an extreme where you won't eat out or eat any type of food unless it is organic, natural and unprocessed can become mentally draining and lead to obsession.

If you cannot remember the last time you ate out or even enjoyed your food, you need to loosen the food rules a little. There is nothing wrong with healthy eating but if it's limiting you socially, there is a problem. To break free of this health-obsession, think about what foods you really enjoy eating and make sure you have those included in your meal plan. Practise eating out at new places and making decisions on regular menu items. And most importantly, remember that food is meant to nourish your body and eating is meant to be a pleasurable experience. If you do not find this is the case, you may need to speak to a professional on issues relating to control in your life.

Food habits
that make you fat

*'You have the power and the opportunity
to change your habits.'*

It is not the one-off trip to your favourite fast-food shop or bakery that results in you carrying extra weight – it's the extra calories that slip in on a daily basis because of the poor food habits you've developed over time. The extra coffee at work, eating the kids' leftovers or enjoying a high-calorie treat every night after dinner... The first step towards kicking bad food habits is to identify them. When do you notice yourself eating something not because you are hungry but because it is there? When do you look forward to a food reward throughout the day? Here are some of the most common poor food habits.

EATING IN THE CAR
Eating in the car starts when we're running late, then it becomes something we do every day to save time and before you know it, you find yourself always looking for food when you're behind the wheel.

The link between driving and food means you are more likely to look for a service station to purchase unhealthy snacks and coffees every time you're driving for extended periods. Make a commitment to not eat in the

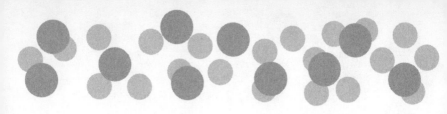

car at all and instead always keep your water bottle and some mints with you for when you need something in your mouth but know you don't need the calories.

EATING IN FRONT OF THE TV

Eating in front of the TV is a terrible habit of modern life. We get home late and reward ourselves with a quick meal in front of our favourite sitcom or DVD. The issue with this is that we're not concentrating on how much we're eating and hence are likely to overeat.

Make a commitment to only eat food sitting down at the table – no excuses. Studies have shown that individuals eat more calories throughout the course of the day when they have eaten meals in front of the TV. Not paying attention to what you're eating affects your ability to self-monitor. If you must, limit it to just once a week, on a Sunday for example, so you are at lower risk of the habit developing again when you're tired. Keep your eating area, such as the kitchen or dining table, clear so it's easy to sit and eat a meal there, and create a nice environment with a candle or music so that you link dinner to feeling relaxed and comfortable, especially if you have small children.

SOMETHING SWEET AT 3 PM

Remember that a strong craving for intense flavour, whether it be sweet or savoury, generally means that your meal beforehand did not contain

enough bulky salad vegetables and/or protein. While eating at 3 pm can become a habit, if there's an underlying physiological reason why you're looking for these flavours at certain times, at some point you need to work out why so you can manage it and ideally prevent the craving.

First check your lunch to make sure that you've included both a good source of protein and salad or vegetables. If you still crave something sweet at 3 pm, try not to wait until the craving is extreme before you eat. Have something savoury first and notice how this takes away your craving for sugar rather than feeding it. Crackers with low-fat cheese or cream cheese are a good choice. Then if you also eat something small and sweet such as a single low-fat cookie, some fresh fruit or a portion-controlled chocolate, you will have also had the savoury food to help regulate your blood glucose levels for the rest of the afternoon.

GORGING BEFORE DINNER

It's common to have an extreme urge to eat when you get home from work as it's been several hours since lunch. The key is to prevent this intense hunger so you're more in control when making your food choice.

The easiest strategy to prevent late-afternoon hunger is to get into a habit of grabbing an apple or carrot to eat on the way home from work. This way you've eaten something healthy and taken the edge off your hunger, so you're less likely to overdo it and spoil your dinner.

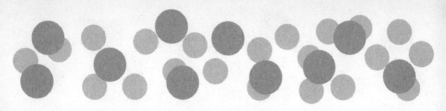

EATING THE KIDS' LEFTOVERS

This is an easy trap for parents to fall into, generally because they prioritise the kids' needs over their own, and because it's easy to pick at food in front of you.

First of all, if you routinely have leftovers from your kids' meals, you are preparing too much food. Get used to putting leftovers in containers immediately to reserve for later so that you're not tempted. Most importantly, prioritise your own food needs so you don't get over-hungry. Remember parents who look after themselves are in a better place mentally and physically to care for their children.

Are your hormones making you fat?

'Insulin resistance is a clinical condition that requires a specific dietary and lifestyle approach.'

For many years, scientists, nutritionists and numerous other weight-loss professionals have preached that weight loss comes down to a very simple equation – calories in versus calories out. While this principle is true to a certain extent, it is a little too simplistic. There are a number of hormonal shifts that can occur to alter this relationship. One such diagnosis is insulin resistance, the clinical condition that precedes type 2 diabetes. Individuals with insulin resistance will struggle to lose weight via traditional weight-loss methods simply because their body is not burning fuel the way it should be.

Insulin is a hormone which is secreted by the pancreas and used to digest carbohydrates. When carbohydrate-rich foods are consumed, insulin is secreted by the pancreas to take glucose from the bloodstream to the muscles for energy. For a number of reasons, over time, insulin may fail to work as well as it should. Weight gain, where fat is clogging the cells, is such a reason, as is a lack of physical activity. Your genetics can also predispose you to insulin resistance and type 2 diabetes. Another significant contributing factor to insulin resistance is the highly processed nature of our daily carb choices including breads, breakfast cereals and

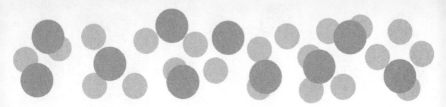

snack foods, which require much higher amounts of insulin than less-processed low-GI carbs.

Resistance to insulin builds up over time, with the body gradually producing more and more insulin to get glucose out of the blood and into the body's cells for energy. As insulin is also a fat-storing hormone, the more of it that's circulating in the body, the harder it becomes to actually burn body fat. High levels of insulin can also make you feel tired and bloated and crave sugar, as the body is not getting the fuel it needs to the cells as efficiently as it should be. Individuals with insulin resistance also tend to have distinct abdominal fat deposits and carry much of their weight around their belly.

Once diagnosed by a physician or endocrinologist, insulin resistance can be managed. Tight management can actually prevent the development of type 2 diabetes. While some cases will warrant medication, the diet and exercise prescription does not change. Individuals with insulin resistance need a reduced carb, increased protein diet developed by a specialist dietitian, as well as a highly specific training program that integrates high-intensity cardio sessions in conjunction with a light resistance-training program. Individuals with insulin resistance need to learn to become extremely fussy with their choice of carbs. High-GI carbs, including juice, white bread and refined cereals, need to be completely eliminated from the diet for the best weight-loss outcomes long-term.

Signs that you may have a degree of insulin resistance that may be worth investigating include an inability to lose weight despite a healthy diet and exercise routine, distinct abdominal fat, feeling unusually fatigued, bloated and craving sugar regularly. Identifying insulin resistance early and committing to a 6–12 month diet and exercise intervention may help you avoid getting diabetes.

So if you are a veteran of the weight-loss industry and cannot seem to lose weight no matter which diet you try, it may be time for a trip to your doctor for a glucose tolerance test (with insulin levels) to be performed after you have eaten a high-carb diet for 3 days. The test will check how your hormones are responding to sugar when it's present in your blood. High insulin levels on this test indicate that your hormones are working too hard to maintain an optimal blood glucose level, which will fast track you to type 2 diabetes if not managed.

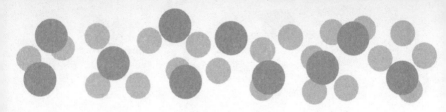

Reset your hunger switch

'When was the last time you felt really, really hungry?'

Although hunger is the primary physiological cue to tell us that we need more food, very few of us eat solely according to our hunger signals. We eat because food is in front of us, because it is a meal or snack time, because we're bored or because we're scared that we might get hungry later.

Failing to eat according to hunger over long periods of time means that we are at risk of constantly overeating, and hence making our food choices externally rather than internally driven. This means we eat more and more, and program our belly and head into thinking we need more food than we actually do. If you cannot remember the last time you actually felt really hungry, it's time to reset your hunger. Ideally we need to feel hungry every 2–3 hours. Hunger is a sign that you're burning your food well. It is a sign that your metabolism is working optimally.

Often people who eat too much at night don't wake up hungry and then skip breakfast. Such a behavioural pattern is not only shifting your caloric intake towards the second half of the day, but means that you're skipping your early morning hunger signal. Some claim they don't eat breakfast

because it actually makes them hungrier throughout the morning. But such regular hunger is a good thing, it's a sign a dormant metabolism is kicking in.

To reset your hunger switch, try having a very light meal at 5 or 6 pm for your dinner. Good options include a vegetable soup (see recipe on the following page) or some sushi. Then wait at least 12–14 hours until you eat a large breakfast of eggs on toast or Bircher muesli the next morning. Not only should you be hungry for this meal, but you should be satisfied until midmorning when you need to eat something that will again fill you for 2–3 hours.

If you actually feel nauseous in the mornings and really cannot tolerate anything, start reintroducing breakfast slowly. Remember that your body has not been used to eating so early for some time so it will take time to reprogram it. Start with a small snack first thing such as a couple of plain crackers. Over time you will notice your morning appetite improves as long as you keep your evening meal light and enjoy it by 8 pm.

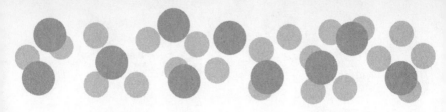

ROAST VEGETABLE SOUP

1 capsicum, chopped roughly

2 carrots, chopped roughly

1 parsnip, chopped roughly

2 onions, halved

500 g pumpkin, chopped roughly

350 g sweet potato, chopped roughly

4 cloves of garlic

750 ml gluten-free vegetable stock

¼ cup light sour cream

fresh thyme

Serves 4–6

1 Preheat oven to 180°C. Place the vegetables on a large baking tray and brush them lightly with olive oil. Bake for an hour, turning occasionally.

2 Remove the capsicum, but continue to bake the other vegetables for a further 30 minutes.

3 Once the capsicum is cooled, remove the skin (this should rub off easily) and blend with the carrot, parsnip and onion.

4 Add in the pumpkin, sweet potato, garlic and half the stock – purée until smooth.

5 Put everything in a pan with the remaining stock and heat through. Serve with a ¼ cup of sour cream on top and sprinkle with fresh thyme.

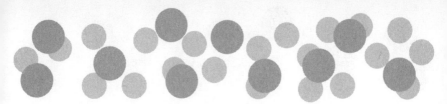

Consider a fast

'Intermittent fasting appears to offer many benefits, from both a metabolic and weight-control perspective.'

The first thing to know when it comes to fasting is that it is not a new concept. Individual cultures and religions have embraced fasting for hundreds of years, both for spiritual reasons and for its physical benefits. From a dietary perspective, significant research into the physiological benefits of fasting can be traced back to the 1930s, when researchers identified that rats fed significant fewer calories not only lived much longer, but had much lower rates of cancer.

In recent years the concept of regular fasting has gained significant attention off the back of the work of British scientist Dr Michael Mosely, who authored *The 5:2 Diet*. Mosely's approach is to incorporate two non-consecutive days of very low-calorie eating (just 500–600 calories or ¼ of your regular calorie intake), followed by five days of regular, non-restrictive eating. Since the release of this diet there have been a number of variations to the 5:2 model. An alternative program suggests limiting food consumption to just 8 hours of every day; another advises not eating until lunchtime, therefore supporting a prolonged overnight fast, or limiting food consumption to just one meal per day. Each of these variations – depending on compliance – potentially offer benefits.

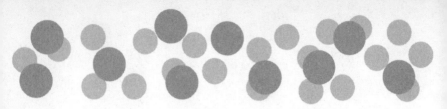

Research suggests that any prolonged period without eating, or eating very few calories for short periods, supports lower cholesterol, blood pressure and blood glucose control.

The most important thing to consider when it comes to fasting is what will be the most sustainable dietary option for you. All diets work, but the issue is that many people cannot stick to them. In the case of fasting, both a 5:2 or extended overnight fast will have metabolic benefits and support weight control. However, if you can't stick to an especially low-calorie diet, or hunger is likely to get the better of you if you do not eat for several hours, fasting may not be the right approach for you.

If you have no issue sticking to strict regimes, the choice is between fasting via a couple of specific low-calorie days or for extended periods of the day, every day. In the case of a 5:2 approach, this means sticking to just 500–600 calories, which in food terms translates to just two meals (for example, one poached egg with a cup of vegetables and a piccolo coffee in one meal and just 80–100 g fish and vegetables or salad in the other). For non-eaters, such as busy businessmen or shift workers, this may not seem that extreme, but for the average person, who tends to eat several times a day, such an enormous shift in eating habits may not prove that easy, particularly in social situations. In my experience followers tend to eat more like 800–1000 calories per day while fasting – often an extra coffee or snack slips in, which, unfortunately, negates the benefits of the 'fast'.

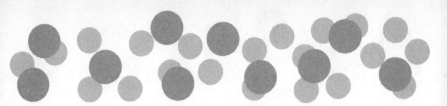

If such severe calorie restriction is not for you, another option is to simply limit the number of hours you consume food each day. For example, eating only between 8 am and 4 pm or 10 am and 6 pm. In these examples, while you are not limiting calories to an extreme level, you are allowing an extended period of time for the body's hormones to return to baseline levels without constantly being disrupted with numerous feeding occasions. While research examining this exact approach is limited, any regime that limits calorie intake via clear daily structure is likely to support weight loss.

Ultimately the key component of any fasting approach to dieting is compliance and consistency. We know that there are a number of health benefits, but it comes down to deciding what is the right way to incorporate this style of eating into your lifestyle without the feelings of deprivation that can come from extreme dieting.

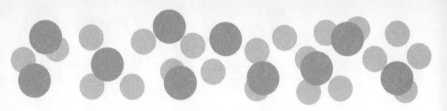

Mindless munching

'When we eat mindfully, we eat less and enjoy our food more. Eat slowly, chew your food, savour.'

Since the term 'mindless eating' was explored in depth by eating behaviour researcher Brian Wansink, more attention has been paid to not only what we eat but the way we do it. Mindless eating occurs when we're not paying attention – a handful of jelly beans, a couple of bites of the kids' leftovers, the pre-dinner snack of cheese and crackers while you chop the vegetables. When we're not paying attention to what goes in our mouths, we're likely to eat far more than we need, to not register that we've eaten it and to fail to compensate at our next meal. Being more mindful about the way we eat is crucial in avoiding extra calories slipping into our day, resulting in extra weight gain long-term.

Mindless eating occurs when you're distracted or doing something else. Eating when driving, watching TV or preparing dinner, for example. It can easily become a habit when you naturally link a certain situation to eating – grabbing a chocolate bar when filling the car with petrol or saying yes to coffee and cake by default when meeting friends.

To gain control of this type of mindless eating, keep a record of the times food is entering your mouth and then ask yourself, 'Am I hungry, or is eating that food at that time just a bad habit?' Once you recognise when you're eating out of habit, the easier it will be to stop yourself.

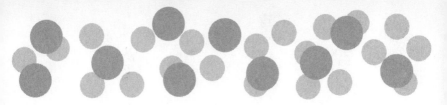

The next step in controlling mindless eating is to limit the amount of food you have around you. Rid your home, office and social environments of as much visible food stimulus as you can. It is time to clear the desk or bench of snacks, the office kitchen of the visible biscuit jar and the car of hidden snacks. Not having food in front of you all the time will make you less likely to think about it outside of meal times. You will start eating out of hunger, rather than in response to visual stimulus.

Mindless eating also occurs when we eat too quickly. Too often we find ourselves rushing to get a meal down so we can move on to our next task. It takes the stomach at least 20 minutes to register that it's had enough food, which is often a few hundred calories after we put the fork down. Recent research has found that diners who were told to chew each mouthful of food at least 20 times, in addition to placing their knife and fork down in between mouthfuls, consumed 20 per cent fewer calories during a meal than those given no such instructions.

Simply being more aware of the need to slow down will naturally see you take more time with each mouthful and each meal. Chew each mouthful carefully and practise placing your knife and fork down in between each mouthful. Aim to always be the last to finish your meal and take a sip of water in between mouthfuls. Cutting your food into smaller pieces also helps to draw the meal out. Finally, always allow a decent amount of time to pass between courses. You'll find you can only eat a couple of mouthfuls of a dessert when you have really let your food settle, as opposed to the whole serve if you eat it immediately after your meal.

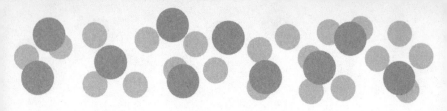

Eating mindfully requires you to concentrate on your food. This means savouring each mouthful, chewing it properly and focusing solely on the eating experience. Being more aware of how much you've eaten will put you in a better position to regulate your energy intake.

Mindless eating traps to avoid

- In the car
- In front of the TV
- In front of the computer
- While reading
- At the desk
- At the kitchen bench
- When preparing dinner

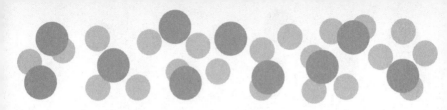

Develop your self-regulation skills

'In a world of food opportunities, self-regulation is what differentiates those who control their weight from those who don't.'

You know how there are the people who can eat half a chocolate bar and leave the rest, or decline offers of dessert no matter how appealing it looks? Or who can skip dinner when they've eaten too much at lunch? Such people have extremely good self-regulatory skills, which will serve them well in many facets of their life, including weight control.

Self-regulation refers to the way in which an individual is able to use self-monitoring and feedback to plan, guide and maintain changes in behaviour to successfully reach their goals. Some aspects of self-regulation are likely to be innate, governed by such physiological signals as hunger and satiety while others are taught to us by parents and other social influencers.

The most primitive of food related self-regulatory variables – hunger and satiety – are innate. Babies, for example, are very good at telling their mothers when they are hungry and when they have had enough. But the rapidly growing rate of obesity suggests that these cues are easily overridden. We all know it's easy to overeat, yet not so easy to skip a meal.

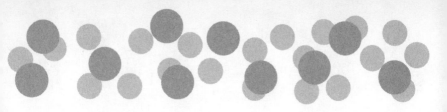

It's easy to allow one drink to turn into four, or a few pieces of chocolate to become an entire block. Such programmed behaviour is easy to repeat time and time again when it is all we have ever known. In such instances, food is not being consumed because of taste or desire but rather as instant reward and part of a learnt habit.

We each have a different required level of self-regulation that will allow us to control our food intake and our weight. For example, some of us will self-regulate by eating well during the week while relaxing things a little at weekends, while others will judge the degree of self-regulation required by keeping an eye on the scales or belt notches to determine when things appear to be creeping up.

If you know that you lack self-regulatory skills, the first step towards improving them is to determine where they are most lacking. Is it when you drink alcohol? When you are alone at home or when you are eating with friends? Once you are more aware of where your self-regulation abilities are lacking (exercise, food behaviours or both), you are in a position to improve your skills – to be able to clearly state that you will only be having two drinks or that you will skip the chips with your meal. Once you have one or two self-regulatory strategies you will be in a much better position to start to govern the rules around these cues. As is the case with any new habit, practice will be required in order for these skills to translate into normal behaviour. The good news is that 3 months after a new behaviour is adopted, you will find that you no longer need to think about it – the healthy decision will come naturally.

Build your willpower

'Like a muscle, willpower can be practised and built over time.'

Willpower – the ability to hold back when you need to; to not eat the entire block of chocolate; to go to the gym even when you are tired; to not stop at the fast-food drive-through even though you really, really want to – is a term we often hear about in motivational literature. Some individuals appear to naturally have endless buckets of the stuff – the buffed personal trainers who never let a skerrick of junk food pass their lips or the resolute dieter who can starve their body for months and months at a time. Despite the fact that this way of being can seem to be innate, it appears the way we think about our ability to exert willpower is is in fact the most powerful aspect of self-control.

Early behavioural research exploring young children's ability to exercise willpower and delay gratification was researched in the late 1960s and 1970s by psychologist Walter Mishel from Stanford University. The studies found that the largely innate ability of 4-year-olds to delay gratification (not eat the marshmallow) for reward (two marshmallows instead of one) predicted success across a range of life domains 20 years later.

Recently, our glucose levels have been identified as another significant factor in our ability to exercise willpower. Specifically, lab based research studies have shown that some factors associated with the ability to

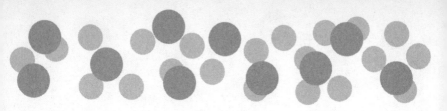

exercise willpower – attention, emotional regulation and suppression – are impaired when blood glucose levels are lowered. When this is considered in a dieting context, it suggests that fluctuating blood glucose levels caused by dietary restriction of calories and/or carbohydrates may directly impair one's ability to exercise willpower.

More recently, research has found that it is primarily the beliefs we hold about our ability to demonstrate willpower that impact our ability to maintain self-control and focus. A study published in the journal *Proceedings of the National Academy of Sciences* explained the results of an experiment where individuals who believed that their willpower was abundant did not need the extra sugar they were offered to help them complete challenging tasks, whereas the participants who believed their willpower was limited did better after they had consumed a sugary drink. These findings would suggest that your beliefs about your own willpower are something to think about if you are finding self-control challenging.

So if you naturally struggle with maintaining your own willpower, here are some simple strategies that may help you to build your willpower muscle, rather than letting it control you.

1. SLOW DOWN

Fast, mindless eating leaves us prone to overeating and poor decision making. This is especially true for individuals who innately seek out self-gratification without considering the consequences, or the fast drinker or eater who always finishes their meal first. The simple act of pacing – taking time to make considered food and drink choices and then mindfully eating and drinking over longer periods of time – naturally helps you to practise self-control.

2. KEEP YOUR BLOOD GLUCOSE LEVELS STABLE

We are much more likely to make poor food decisions when our blood glucose levels are low. This may be due to poor diet, unstructured meals and snacks, high intake of caffeine, or sugar from lollies and soft drinks throughout the day. Regular meals every 3–4 hours that contain both carbohydrates and proteins will support optimal blood glucose regulation.

3. BUILD YOUR BELIEFS

Recent research suggests that if you think you can do it, you probably can, but if you think you need extra treats and sugars to get you through, you will. Practise positive self-talk to program your natural thought patterns to focus on what you can do, and how you are going to achieve it, rather than looking for reasons and excuses not to.

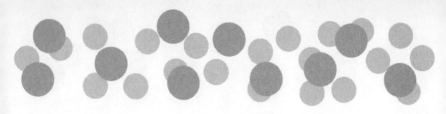

4. DO NOT LEAVE YOURSELF VULNERABLE

If you struggle to control your food impulses, try to control your environment so you are not vulnerable. Stop buying the food you do not want to eat. Avoid cooking too much and consuming extra portions. Often we are our own worst enemies when it comes to controlling our food intake.

5. KNOW YOUR HIGH RISK FOODS AND SCENARIOS

You may be prone to overeating at night, or a 3 pm sugar binge. Or you may hate the gym, or exercising in the afternoon. The best thing you can do to stay on top of these risky times is to actively manage them, rather than waiting to become a victim of them. This may mean scheduling activities in the evening or seeking out another approach to training. Put simply, if you really want to change your diet and lifestyle choices, you need to actively take steps to change your behavioural patterns.

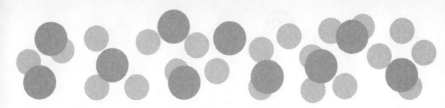

Managing cravings

'You never need to be a victim to your cravings.'

Many people are victims of their food cravings. They fight the desire for salty, sweet or fatty foods until they can no longer manage the mental battle and completely give in, generally eating much more than they need to feel satisfied.

Food cravings actually give us valuable information about what is going on in our bodies. For example, craving sweet foods late in the afternoon generally means that you haven't eaten enough protein and/or salad with your lunch and need to refuel. A craving can also be the result of programming the body to look for certain taste sensations at certain times of day. If you always eat a biscuit with your morning coffee, your brain is going to be looking for a biscuit every day at 10 am until you break the association.

Physiological cravings are completely within your control. A significant drop in blood glucose levels (which can occur when uneven amounts of carbohydrates are consumed throughout the day) is the most common reason we crave sugar. If you go without carbs or choose the wrong types, you leave yourself vulnerable to extreme sugar highs and lows. Simply aim to eat a slowly digested, low-GI carb every 3–4 hours, even in very small amounts, to help support optimal blood glucose regulation and prevent sugar cravings.

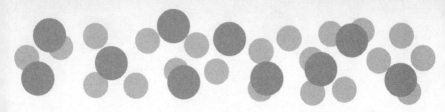

Behavioural cravings can be curbed by breaking the association between food and certain times of the day. Breaking the link by going cold turkey on the food you crave is ideal, but a more gentle craving management plan is to first just delay the craving. Rather than instantly eating the food you crave, try and have at least 10 minutes doing something else. You'll be surprised how many times you can eliminate this need for sugar or fat by simply slowing down the eating process and reconsidering. A recent study found that a significant number of participants lost their craving for chocolate when they had to go for a walk before they were allowed to indulge the craving.

Most of the time you just need to change the taste in your mouth. Green tea or iced water with a lemon slice are great ways to kill a craving for sugar, as is sugar-free gum and mints. Brushing your teeth is also a proven technique to quell cravings.

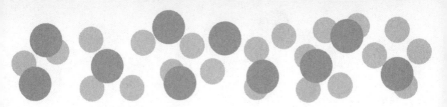

Learn to stop overeating

*'Just as you have taught yourself to overeat,
you can teach yourself not to.'*

We all eat high-calorie, high-fat foods from time to time and have
periods where we overeat, whether due to boredom, celebration,
comfort or not having the ability to clearly identify hunger. If indulgence
happens occasionally at celebrations and parties it's not such an issue.
For those of us who find ourselves overeating regularly and gaining
weight as a result, it's time to take a closer look at why the overeating
is occurring.

Overeating is extremely easy because the body lets it happen. If fullness
was anywhere near as strong a sensation as hunger, few of us would have
issues regulating the volume of food we eat. If it's been some time since
you have managed to stop eating at the right time, it's time to get back in
touch with your body's natural appetite signals. Signs that you may be
overdoing it on a regular basis include not feeling hungry, being able to
eat much larger volumes of food than you had previously and, of course,
your clothes getting tighter.

Try serving yourself much smaller portions, even half of your regular
meal if you have to, and eat as slowly as possible. Try ending the meal
a mouthful or so before you usually would to remind yourself of what
feeling comfortably full feels like. Such a process will take time – weeks or

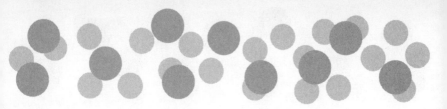

even months – but it's important to work through it to remind yourself of the body's natural hunger and satiety signals.

The most important thing to do if you or other family members are prone to overeating is to limit the type and volume of food that is kept in the home. Forget the idea of having a chocolate stash in your desk that you'll only raid in emergencies or keeping a packet of biscuits in the cupboard that you'll only open if guests visit, because if it's there you will eat it.

Another strategy to implement as you seek to gain control is to compensate when you do overindulge. Learning to balance indulgences rather than trying to avoid them altogether is the key to weight control success. This simply means that if you've overdone it for a meal, make sure you cut back on the next. Longer periods of indulgence in turn need longer periods of compensation. A week of holiday eating equals a week of eating lightly.

The best light options to balance your diet during these periods of lighter eating include vegetable-based juice, broth-style soups, meal-replacement shakes and salads. The secret to compensating well is to not let yourself starve. As soon as you are starving (either psychologically with small volumes of food or literally with inadequate nutrition), the more difficult it will be to stay on track with your lighter diet. Instead, leave your diet with the same volume of food but with fewer calories.

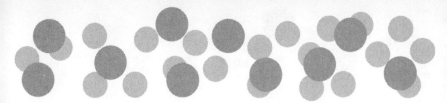

Top 10 tips to avoid overeating

1   Plan your meals and snacks so you don't get too hungry and prone to overeating.
2   Avoid buffets.
3   Put leftovers away before you sit down to eat your meal.
4   Eat lightly during the day if you're going out for dinner.
5   End your meal with something small and sweet.
6   Go for a walk after meals to get out of the kitchen.
7   Don't over shop. Buy only what you need each week.
8   Have a snack before you attend social occasions where food will be served.
9   Quantify your hunger and aim to only eat when you are at 8–9 out of 10.
10 Chew gum or brush your teeth after meals.

Think thin

'Thin people most likely eat less and exercise more than you do.'

Chances are you have a friend, family member or colleague who seems to effortlessly control their weight while you gain a kilogram even thinking about a slice of cake. What is it that these individuals do differently to the rest of us? Well, it appears that there are a number of lifestyle habits and commonalities among these individuals that the rest of us can learn from.

THEY DO NOT 'DIET'

Forget detoxing, or juice fasts, or the latest diet regime. Evidence suggests that slim people consume a basic healthy diet that eliminates nothing but seeks balance with everything. The issue with diets is that they tend to immediately elicit a feeling of deprivation, which can lead to excessive focus on food and eating, fuelling binges and food obsessions which negate any benefits associated with the original diet. The take-home message here is that if a diet feels restrictive, it is unlikely to help you with weight control long-term.

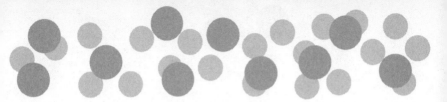

THEY EXERCISE, A LOT

Evidence available suggests that individuals who lose weight and keep it off exercise for at least an hour each day, and those who are naturally slim work out at least five days per week. Calorie-wise this equates to a 2000 plus calorie burn every single week, or the equivalent of more than a day's worth of calories.

THEY EAT VEGETABLES, A LOT OF THEM

No surprises here. Dietary regimes shown to have long-term health benefits include the Mediterranean diet and the DASH diet, which include 7–10 serves (3½ to 5 cups) of fresh fruit and vegetables every single day! It makes sense: when you eat this much fresh produce, there is far less room for high-calorie foods.

THEY THINK QUALITY OVER QUANTITY

This is a big one. Long-term weight control is not about focusing on what you should not eat, rather it is about enjoying good quality food, high calorie or not. It means not wasting calories on the mindless extras that slip into our diets without us realising. The extra snacks and fast food that we do not necessarily enjoy can add hundreds of calories to our regular intake. It means enjoying a small serve of good quality cake rather than eating an entire packet of biscuits for the sake of it. Or a glass or two of great wine rather than a whole bottle of cheap or free grog. It is about asking the question, 'Is this really worth the calories?'

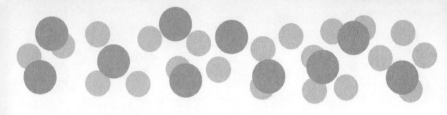

THEY SHOP SMART

One of the easiest ways to examine diet quality is to inspect your grocery bill. If it is minus the processed, packaged snacks and high-fat treats it is a good sign. However, if you regularly purchase foods you know you shouldn't, you have lost the battle. If you buy them, you are eating them. If you know you should not eat them for weight control, you need to get honest and stop buying them.

THEY COOK AT HOME

Meals prepared at home have significantly fewer calories than meals we purchase away from the home. For example, popular lunch choices at the food court contain almost double the calories of the comparable meal you prepare for yourself. Restaurant meals can contain an entire day's worth of calories. For this reason, simply cooking at home more often is an easy step towards weight control.

THEY KEEP THEIR DIET STABLE

It does not matter if it is Christmas, a major birthday, winter – individuals who control their weight maintain diet structure. There is no such thing as taking a week off their diet: they might enjoy a one-off heavy meal or the occasional treat, but will always resume their normal diet straight after.

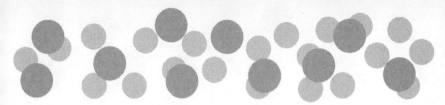

THEY SNACK SMART

Forget packaged snacks, low-fat treats and processed foods: snacking means something light and nutritious for those in control of their weight. Fruit, nuts and dairy are all nutrient-rich, calorie controlled, natural food options that represent a good snack in calorie terms. (Snacks should not be a mini meal.)

THEY DON'T DO FOOD GUILT

Forget diet talk and cycles of deprivation and binging. Food is not used to soothe emotional states and there is an understanding that at times we will overindulge and consume higher fat, higher calorie foods but it all evens out eventually. There is no guilt, nor compensatory behaviours associated with eating: it is about good habits, occasional treats and that boring concept of balance.

THEY KEEP AN EYE ON THEIR WEIGHT

Individuals who control their weight frequently report weighing themselves regularly. Not only does regular weighing mean that you notice when the scales are creeping up, but you can also respond quickly and take the steps required to reverse weight gain, before it becomes significant.

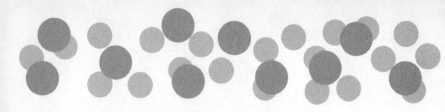

Expect a plateau

'Plateaus are part of the weight-loss process and should be expected.'

A common weight-loss scenario is to have an initial successful weight loss of 3–5 kg after some diet modification, then nothing. Nothing happens on the scales for a couple of weeks and sometimes your weight may even increase by a few hundred grams. Why does this happen and how can you move yourself off the dreaded weight-loss plateau?

Weight-loss plateaus occur for a very simple reason. The human body likes to be stable and doesn't like losing weight. Once it has lost weight it works better, we know this, but the body perceives weight loss as a negative energy state and will do everything it can to halt this loss. If the body thinks it is receiving too few calories or if weight has been lost rapidly, the metabolism may in fact be slowed in order to conserve energy. This is the most common reason weight loss slows down when food intake has been reduced for extended periods of time.

There are several strategies that can be implemented to move you out of a weight-loss plateau. Ironically, in many cases you may have to eat a little more. Following a very low-calorie or low-carbohydrate food plan for extended periods of time may have pushed the metabolism to breaking point. So to kickstart things, try increasing your calories slightly – just

100–200 extra each day by increasing the size of your breakfast or lunch while still keeping your energy intake low during the second half of the day. Another option is to keep your diet strict during the first half of the week before relaxing a little over the weekend and enjoying larger meals or the alcohol or dessert you've been skipping.

Other tricks to try include eating breakfast earlier, as well as alternating the size of your breakfast, aiming to be hungry by midmorning. Not experiencing hunger may mean that your meals are being consumed too late in the day or are too large. Your breakfast should keep you full for 2–3 hours. If you are hungry after an hour, your breakfast does not have the right balance of protein and carbs. Try changing your breakfast choice to be hungry for a light snack midmorning. This means your body is burning its food well and your metabolism is firing up.

Finally, remember to check your training intensity. Training before breakfast can be a great way to get the metabolism moving. The same goes for changing the type and duration of your regular training. Keeping your body guessing is the answer to both getting off a weight-loss plateau and kickstarting your metabolic rate.

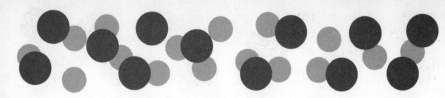

your BODY

'The sooner you accept that you need to move your body every day, the sooner you'll be able to focus your energy on finding a training plan that works for you.'

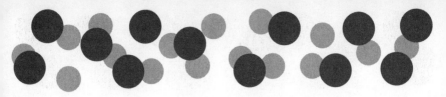

Start small   182

Measure your body   184

Get a pedometer   186

Start training   188

Learn to interval train   190

Time to lift   191

Check your calories   193

Fuel your body for training   198

Is working out making
    you fatter?   201

Start small

'There's no point starting an ambitious gym routine and only getting through one week – build your training regime gradually.'

If you want to enjoy your favourite foods while controlling your weight, you need to exercise regularly. We know that exercise is good for us for a myriad of reasons but we also know that busy lifestyles may not always be conducive to regular workouts, particularly if exercise has never been a priority in your life.

The beautiful thing about exercise is that if done the right way, at the right time, it teaches your body to burn food better. The better your body is able to burn, the more food you will be able to eat. For the majority of us who really like to eat, this can only be a good thing. But if exercise isn't done regularly or effectively, it may leave you prone to hunger and over-compensation, and in exactly the same place weight-wise.

The rule of thumb for those beginning to incorporate regular exercise into their lives is to start gently. Rather than committing to five or six sessions a week right away, only to give up completely a week or two later because it's too hard, start with one session each week. The key to success with any new routine is to ensure you choose an activity that you like and is easy for you to do, and schedule it for a day and time when few distractions will come up. As soon as a commitment becomes complex – involving

commutes, traffic, children, work finishing on time or an activity you are not that keen on, the chances that you will get there decrease significantly.

The easiest option by far is to walk for just 20–30 minutes first thing in the morning. A small time commitment is less likely to be overwhelming, you can get it out of the way before you start your day and no matter what fitness level you are at, you can manage it. Remember that a walk you do once a week, every week for the rest of your life is going to be much better than a gym class you do for 2 weeks and never again. Start small and build – the easier it fits into your already chaotic schedule, the better.

Top 10 easy ways to move more

1 Get off the bus or the train a stop earlier.
2 Park as far away from your destination as you can.
3 Use the bathroom on a different level in the office.
4 Always take the stairs.
5 If there are no stairs, walk up escalators.
6 Get out and run errands every lunchtime.
7 Stand up at least every hour at work.
8 If you have a question for someone in the office, go and ask them in person rather than sending an email.
9 Always volunteer to pick up the coffees.
10 Walk after dinner.

Measure your body

'Measurements tell us more about the health of our body than our weight ever will.'

Are you terrified of the scales? Would you rather die than have to get on the scales in front of other people? It is safe to say, you are not alone. Scale phobias have often been developed at a young age stemming from uncomfortable memories of a doctor's appointment or gym class when our weight was exposed for all to see, and of course it was a weight that was much higher than we would have liked.

While body weight can be used as a rough marker of health and fitness, for anyone who trains regularly, body composition is a much more insightful marker of health and a more accurate measure of body fat. If you are 90 kg and should be 70 kg, there is no doubt that you want to see reductions on the scales over time. But if you are 65 kg and want to be 60 kg, and your body weight doesn't change but your measurements decrease significantly, it is still an excellent weight-loss outcome. This means you're losing body fat while maintaining muscle mass.

Solely judging your weight loss outcome on shifting scale readings, especially when we're dealing with relatively small amounts of body

weight, is almost certainly setting yourself up to fail. You need to take body measurements as well as weight to really monitor how your body is changing. For men, a simple waist measurement is all you need, while women can benefit from a waist, hip, bust and bottom measurement. Never weigh or measure yourself more than once each week, as body weight and size can differ by as much as 1–2 kg over the course of the day. Always take your measurements first thing in the morning and remember that if you have a salty meal the night before you take the measurements, your weight may be up as much as 1–2 kg thanks to the fluid retention your body encourages to balance out the extra salt.

For the scale addicts out there who weigh themselves multiple times per week, or even per day, this behaviour is likely to be keeping weight on. Psychologically, not seeing positive progress can often reinforce the desire to go off track with the mentality, 'well it's not working anyway'. People with this level of weight-loss obsession need to be banned from the scales for at least a month and then limited to weighing and measuring at most once each week to regain some perspective. Your focus should be on your general health and fitness, not a number.

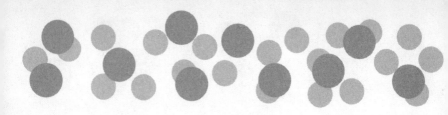

Get a pedometer

*'It's not just the time you spend on the treadmill,
but what you do in between.'*

Do you know how many steps you walk each day? Not on the treadmill
or with your running group, but as part of your daily routine? If you have
no idea, it is time to invest in a wonderful little gadget called a pedometer.

An adult needs to take at least 10,000 steps a day just to maintain their
weight. If you want to actually lose weight, you need to bump that
number right up to 12,000–20,000. To give you some idea of the distance
and time you have to travel to clock up these numbers, you are looking
at about an hour for every 7500–10,000 steps. The average office worker
who drives to and from work will be lucky to manage 2000 steps each day.
No wonder many of us feel tired, bloated and just uncomfortable as we sit
and constrict our digestive organs.

A great lifestyle habit you start making today is to go for a 20–30-
minute walk after dinner, rather than sitting down, leaving your full
belly compacted, bloated and uncomfortable. What do you usually
do after your evening meal? Sit on the couch and watch TV? Clean
up the kitchen? Collapse into bed? Eat chocolate with a cup of tea?
An evening walk not only creates a fantastic time window for families

to communicate without the distractions of TV and computers but it also has a great effect on gut comfort and digestion. Your food will have a chance to settle and move through the digestive tract and leave you feeling lighter and more likely to sleep better as a result.

It's routine that sees us develop and maintain healthy lifestyles. Exercising needs to become the same as brushing our teeth before we get into bed or clearing the table after we eat a meal – automatic.

MOVEMENT	CALORIES BURNT PER DAY	WEIGHT LOSS OVER A YEAR (kg)
Using a bathroom on a different level of your office building	120	4
Getting off public transport a stop early	100	3.5
Walking a flight of stairs each hour	64	2
Getting up every hour and moving for 2 minutes	48	1.5
Getting up to do a chore each ad break when watching TV	36	2

Start training

'Walking's good but on its own it's not enough – you have to train.'

It is not uncommon to hear clients describe proudly how they managed to squeeze a 20- or 30-minute walk into their frantic schedule. It may come as a surprise but the human body was built to move a lot, every day. The endless sitting in front of the computer, TV and steering wheel are in fact the exact opposite of the body's design plan, and we have a growing list of lifestyle-related diseases that demonstrate its unhappiness with our sedentary lifestyle. So as we pat ourselves on the back for walking around the block or completing a few minutes on the treadmill, we are really just making up for part of the time we've spent sitting.

While walking will help burn the calories you have ingested over the day and keep your muscles active and burning, to actually lose weight and keep the muscles working at their best, they need to be trained. Training, as opposed to walking, requires your muscles to be stressed, your heart rate to be high and your blood to be pumping. This challenges every cell to burn more fuel and, as a result, improves fitness and cell function. Such training will keep the body at its best rather than simply preventing it from further age-related decline.

But don't be scared – training doesn't mean spending hours inside a hot, sweaty gym. If you're already walking every day, training can simply

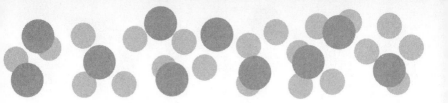

equate to three or four high-intensity cardio sessions for 20–30 minutes each week: a quick workout on the cross trainer, some interval work on the treadmill and a jog instead of a walk. Focusing on quality rather than quantity when it comes to your training means it won't be such a burden on your already full schedule. You can fit a 20–30 minute workout easily into your lunch break, children's sporting classes or before breakfast. A very simple rule that may help you keep on track when it comes to exercise intensity is that if you are not hot and sweaty at the end of the session, you have not been working hard enough.

Top 10 tips for regular exercise

1 Schedule your training sessions at the start of each week.

2 Prioritise your training sessions.

3 Choose exercise that you enjoy.

4 Don't overcommit to exercise.

5 Don't fall off the wagon entirely if you miss a session.

6 Change your sessions regularly.

7 Move as much as you can every day.

8 Exercise to nurture, not torture, your body.

9 Think quality over quantity when it comes to training.

10 Accept that exercise is something that you will have to do forever.

Learn to interval train

'If you are reading a magazine on the exercise bike, you are not pedalling hard enough.'

If you take a look around any gym floor during peak times, I would estimate that 50 per cent of gym users at most are exercising efficiently. Some are watching TV, others reading books or magazines while on their machine. In most cases, these people could and should be burning a lot more calories.

Once you've reached a good level of fitness, interval training is the best way to train efficiently. This means altering the intensity of training at 1-minute intervals to challenge yourself every workout. For the die-hard treadmill fans, this means increasing the incline; for the bike lovers it means turning up the resistance. If you train outdoors the same principle applies – run in between lampposts or seek out some hills. Anything that changes your heart rate and challenges your body will benefit your weight loss and metabolism long-term.

If you consider that you burn more calories in 20 minutes of solid interval training than you do in 40 minutes of regular cardio training, you can see the benefits from both a time management and energy output perspective. Ideally we need to be burning 80–100 calories per 10 minutes to be able to say that we've had a decent workout.

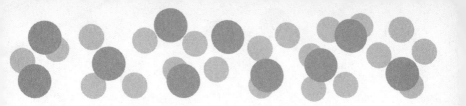

Time to lift

'Lifting weights or resistance training is the best way to teach your body to burn calories.'

It's one thing to eat less to lose weight, and another to move more, but if you're really going to get control of your weight once and for all, you need to teach your body to burn its food better by building muscle tissue.

Resistance training refers to any type of training that places weighted stress on the muscle, which requires it to build and strengthen its cells. Basically, the more muscle mass you have, the more calories you burn. In addition to that, the more your muscles are worked, the better they become at burning, meaning they become more efficient at burning the food you eat. As most of us like to eat and want to be able to eat as much as possible, teaching your muscles to burn energy better is a powerful thing you can do to improve your metabolic rate.

Like all training regimes, the type of resistance training you do is crucial. Ideally you want to be stressing the muscle, which means increasing the weight you can lift over time. For those who have never done any form of resistance training, starting with light weights will see the body respond well initially. Circuit-style classes that include light hand weights and supported weight machines tick this box. If you are already fit, more specialised resistance-style programs may be required.

If you feel that you've been training for some time with no results, or doing the same gym class or personal training session for months with no change to your body shape or size, it's time to check if your training program is up to scratch.

The best option is to consult a highly experienced personal trainer or exercise physiologist to develop a program that is exactly right for you. If this isn't an option, make sure that you are increasing the weight you are lifting and/or increasing the number of sets. Generally speaking, women need to do four to five sets of 12–15 repetitions with lighter weights. If you always use supported weight machines, try swapping to free weights. If you usually train at night, swap to morning sessions or if you always train by yourself, try a boot camp style of training for a change. Remember that the body responds well metabolically to change and challenge. If you are already lifting, you are likely to simply need a change of routine. If you have never lifted, your muscles are waiting for a good workout so get out there.

The body will respond well to even one session a week that has a resistance-training component. For the best results, lifting weights either as part of a program or as a specific weights session in the gym, two to three times each week, will see maximum benefit in terms of both body composition and metabolic rate.

Check your calories

*'Too many active people are running on empty
and then wonder why they cannot lose weight.'*

One of the most common diet scenarios I see is individuals, particularly
females, training regularly but eating fewer calories than a bedridden
70-year-old female needs. Once you're training at a high level (at least an
hour each day) you cannot ruthlessly cut calories without your metabolic
rate being negatively affected. In fact, the further you reduce your calories,
the less likely it is that you're going to lose weight. Your body will be
fighting to store any extra fat as it is effectively being starved of nutrients.

Once you are training regularly, the lowest caloric intake you should allow
yourself is no fewer than 1500 calories. If you're training for more than an
hour a day, you need to increase this by at least 100–200 calories for every
extra hour of activity you do. This will ensure you don't compromise your
metabolic rate too greatly because the body will have adequate fuel for
the amount of activity it is required to do.

Another option for those training hard and cutting calories without
results is to actually reduce your training. A break from your regular
training schedule while keeping calories relatively low is sometimes all
you need to give your muscles a break and your body a chance to reboot
and get back in touch with its natural hunger and satiety signals.

Caloric checklist for training

- Am I eating at least 1500 calories each day?
- Am I eating 100–200 calories extra per hour of intense activity?
- Am I eating breakfast early?
- Am I moving as well as training?
- Am I checking my heart rate when training?
- Am I being careful to not over-train?

If you're unsure why your weight isn't changing, make sure you're accurately measuring both your caloric intake as well as your caloric output. Often we're simply not aware of the extra calories slipping in, so keep a diet diary for a few days and enter all the food and drink you consume. There are dietary analysis packages available, such as 'calorieking', but often the simple act of writing everything down will reveal where you're going wrong. In terms of caloric output, the best indirect measure is determined by checking your heart rate while training using a heart rate monitor. As a rough guide, aim for your heart rate to be working at 70–80 per cent of its maximum rate. To calculate this, simply minus your age from 220 and calculate 70–80 per cent of this number. For example, if you are 40 years old, your ideal heart rate for training would be 135–140 bpm (beats per minute). Of course, always check

this with your doctor prior to starting a new exercise regime. Sometimes regular exercisers simply become used to their regime and are not challenging themselves enough to get the changes in body composition they're looking for.

As a last resort, you can use a very low calorie plan for a short period but only if you're prepared to also cut back your training. The most common detox programs will be 1000–1200 calories. At most, try these programs for just a week or two to give your metabolism a shake up without causing a significant drop in metabolic rate or causing your body to break down muscle tissue for energy.

Unfortunately a healthy diet doesn't always result in fat loss – remember that the balance for fat loss needs to be quite specific, especially when you only have a small amount to lose. Compare the two meal plans on the following pages, for example. Both are very healthy in terms of nutrition, but only the second will result in weight loss.

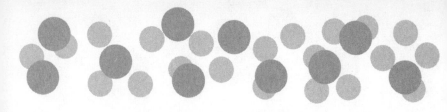

Typical healthy diet

Breakfast	2 large slices of toast with spread
Midmorning snack	2 peaches, 200 g low-fat yoghurt, regular low-fat latte
Lunch	Thai beef stir-fry (no rice)
Pre-dinner snack	Rice crackers, dip, nuts or crackers
Dinner	Chicken stir-fry (no rice)
Dessert	Small bowl of low-fat ice-cream

As you can see, this diet is pretty healthy – the client has even cut carbohydrates at night. But if we analyse the nutrition breakdown:

2200 calories

85 g fat

210 g total carbohydrate

= 45% carbs, 20% protein and 35% fat

= WEIGHT STABLE

While this may look okay, for slow but sustainable fat loss we need to aim for less total calories and an improved ratio of carbs, protein and fat.

Diet for weight loss

Breakfast	2 slices multigrain toast with poached eggs
Midmorning snack	1 peach, 4 grain crackers with 2 slices low-fat cheese, small low-fat latte
Lunch	Grain bread roll (middle removed) with tuna, thin spread avocado and salad
Midafternoon snack	Nut bar, wafer thins with low-fat hommus
Dinner	Thai beef salad
Dessert	Low-fat ice-cream on a stick

The nutrition breakdown is:

> 1600 calories
>
> 60 g fat
>
> 140 g total carbohydrate
>
> = 40% carbs, 30% protein and 30% fat
>
> = FAT LOSS

Despite only small differences, this is the better plan for weight loss.

Fuel your body for training

'Sometimes you need carbs to burn more body fat.'

Sometimes, people who train regularly may struggle to a far greater extent when losing their last bit of weight than those who never train. How can that be?

Regular trainers – those who get up at 5 am every weekday and seriously challenge themselves in each session – are adding stress to a body that is also being denied calories. If a muscle is being trained heavily without enough fuel in the form of carbohydrate, metabolic rate will slow down to protect that muscle. If you have not eaten carbs for a prolonged period, such as an overnight fast of 10–12 hours, and the muscles are then pushed to train for another hour in an intense early-morning workout before breakfast, they are unlikely to be operating at their best metabolically to efficiently burn fat. The same can be said for late-afternoon training sessions when no food has been eaten for 4–5 hours, or since lunch. You are likely to feel tired and lethargic (and hence less

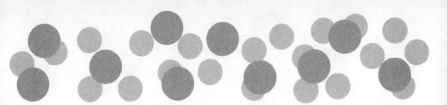

likely to push yourself in the session), but the muscle will simply not have enough fuel to access fat stores effectively.

So if you're already training for a number of hours each week and know that the intensity is there, it may be time to make sure you're giving your muscles the opportunity to burn fat efficiently. If you train pre-breakfast and have chosen to not eat carbs at dinner the night before, try including a small carbohydrate or protein snack before you train. Just a couple of crackers and a slice of low-fat cheese or half a glass of low-fat milk (or the equivalent of 20 g of carbs and 5 g of protein) is all you need.

For those who train midmorning, rather than eating a large breakfast early try halving it, that is one slice of toast or half a bowl of cereal to support maximum fat burning during that session. For afternoon exercisers, make sure you include a protein- or carbohydrate-rich snack 1–2 hours before you train. A nut-based snack bar, some thick yoghurt or a protein shake are all good choices.

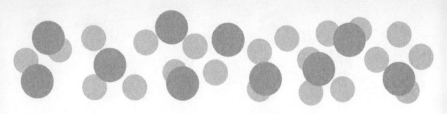

If you haven't eaten carbs at night for years and expect yourself to train for an hour or more every day, it's time to cut your muscles some slack. Try adding ½–1 cup of cooked carbohydrate to your evening meal. Notice how much better you train with a little fuel on board and how much better you feel as a result.

BEST PRE-TRAINING SNACKS	
MORNING	**AFTERNOON**
2 crackers + 1 slice low-fat cheese	Nut-based snack bar
1 slice grain toast + peanut butter	Low-fat milk coffee
½ cup milk	150 g thick yoghurt
½ low-GI muesli bar	4 crackers + 2 slices low-fat cheese
2 tbsp yoghurt	4 corn crackers + peanut butter

Is working out making you fatter?

'It seems the more you exercise, the heavier you get.'

Generally speaking, exercise is a good thing, but in some cases working out can be doing more harm than good. So, if you are exercising more than ever but scales are not moving in the right direction, some of the reasons below could be why.

YOU ARE EATING MORE BECAUSE YOU ARE TRAINING

This is perhaps the most common scenario: we give ourselves permission to eat extra food because we have exercised. An extra banana or small snack should not be an issue, but an extra slice of banana bread, a few biscuits at work or a couple of beers do start to become a problem. Consider your workout the minimum you need to do to keep your weight under control and keep in mind you will need to add in extra if you want to eat more.

YOU ARE EXTRA HUNGRY

If you favour high intensity workouts, such as X-Fit, interval training, cardio sessions of longer than 40–60 minutes, long walks or runs, you may burn a significant number of calories per session – calories the body is keen to make up to keep your weight stable. The end result may be

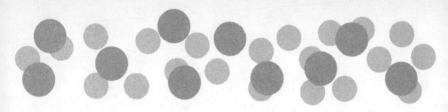

incessant hunger that tends to kick in a few hours after training and lasts all day. There are two options when it comes to managing this: cut back on the amount of time you spend doing these high intensity sessions to just 30–40 minutes or consume a substantial meal immediately after the session in an attempt to take control of the hunger earlier.

YOU ARE NOT TRAINING AS MUCH AS YOU THINK YOU ARE

The amazing thing about the human body is that is adapts very quickly to the stimulus it is exposed to. This means that if you have been doing the same gym routine or run for several months, if not years, chances are you are burning far fewer calories than you think you are. The key to staying on top of metabolic rate is to change things around with both your food and your training every few weeks. Change your running route, get a new weight routine or try some different classes. If in doubt, actively monitor your calorie burn each session with a heart rate or activity monitor – it will offer a more accurate insight into the quality and intensity of your training sessions.

YOU ARE OVEREATING AT NIGHT

Regular exercisers are often disciplined people who have no problem sticking to a strict food regime during the day … before binge eating at night as their body seeks to make up the calorie deficit their training has resulted in. For anyone burning 500–600 calories or more in a single training session – for example a two-hour cycle, X-Fit, run or intense personal training session – you will need an extra meal throughout the

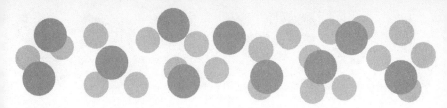

day to help buffer your hunger. This may mean two small lunches instead of one, or morning and afternoon tea. Three meals a day won't cut it if you are regularly burning this many calories.

YOU ARE GIVING YOURSELF PERMISSION TO EAT FOODS YOU NEVER USUALLY WOULD

There is a great sense of entitlement when it comes to eating, and often we think we deserve certain types of food because we have 'been good' or 'earned it'. This seems to be the case especially when it comes to high-fat, high-calorie treats such as cakes, chocolates and desserts that are traditionally saved for special occasions. Just because you have completed five CrossFit workouts or made it to the gym every day does not make it okay to eat extra desserts, cakes or treats. Save those for special occasions and view the gym as part of your regular routine – not a reason to eat more.

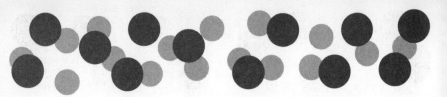

your
LIFE

'Ultimately it's your food, your behaviour,
your body and your life - how do you want
to live it?'

Take control of your office food habits

'Is your office environment conducive to weight control?'

For those of us who spend eight or more hours a day sitting down in an office environment, between the biscuit tin, lolly jar, office lunches and birthday cakes, the calories are literally out to get us. So, if your goal is to keep control of the scales, here are some ways to avoid becoming a victim of workplace weight-gain.

1. BAN THE BISCUITS

You know that once you start, you cannot stop, and while the lure of sugar, fat and white flour can be powerful, there is literally nothing positive you can say about the nutritional profile of plain, sweet biscuits. Perhaps the biggest issue when it comes to the biscuit tin is that once you start to have a biscuit or two with a cup of tea, it quickly becomes a habit and before you know it, you cannot enjoy a hot drink without a biscuit to go with it. Save yourself the heartache and step away from the biscuit tin, for good.

2. STAY AWAY FROM THE FEEDERS

Every office has them, the seemingly well-meaning individuals who make it their job to make sure everyone else eats extra cakes, biscuits and treats they do not really want or need. Sure, there is nothing wrong with making

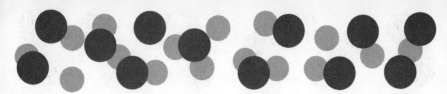

WORK

Take control of your office
    food habits   206

Manage your stress   209

Travel smart   213

HOME

Get a daily timetable   215

Sacred Sunday   217

MOVING FORWARD

You have the power to
    manage your weight   218

Victim no more   219

No more excuses   221

Rejecting laziness   226

See only solutions   227

Commit to self-care   229

Commit to a steely mindset   230

Cement your new habits   232

Maintain your motivation   235

Embrace your true self   237

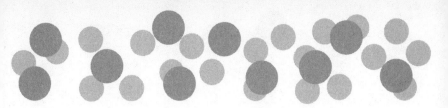

a cake occasionally, but the people who bring in food every other day, organise food-based events and take the chocolate around to everyone's desk at 3 pm can easily sabatage your best intentions. Like the office gossip who you stay wary of, keep well away from the office feeder.

3. GET USED TO TASTING THE CAKE, NOT FINISHING IT

Have you noticed that there is always something to celebrate when you are in the office – a wedding, birthday, someone leaving – which all basically adds up to you eating a whole lot of extra cake. If you struggle to say no when treats and celebratory treats are offered, practise asking for the smallest serve and just tasting the cake. Let's be honest, office cakes are rarely that great that you need to waste your calories on them.

4. BRING YOUR LUNCH

It is really, really hard to find a nutritionally balanced lunch that does not cost the earth. If you are in the habit of treating yourself to fatty, hot meals commonly found in food courts, it is going to be a hard habit to break. The simple act of committing to packing a nutritionally balanced, tasty and filling lunch on most days of the week not only means that you have actively taken control of your nutrition, but it leaves you less vulnerable to emotional ordering. It will also save you money each week. Utilise leftovers, start a work lunch club and, if you really miss your food court lunches, give yourself a treat lunch once each week.

5. SEPARATE WORK AND PLEASURE

Yes, you may spend many, many hours there each week – you may even spend more time with your colleagues than you do your own family – but at the end of the day it is still work. You would not be there if it was not for the pay, and you would not eat half the things you do when you are there if you were at home. There is nothing wrong with enjoying higher calorie treats for special occasions or a few drinks with close friends and family on weekends, but why waste your limited calories at work? The sooner you separate your work and your personal life when it comes to your food and drink decisions, the sooner you will find that it becomes much easier to say no when you know deep down that you should.

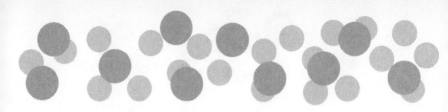

Manage your stress

'Stress is a part of modern life, and managing it is crucial if you want to be at your best.'

Stress – the description given to the feeling of being unable to respond emotionally or physically to real or perceived threats in daily life – appears to be widespread in modern society. Long work hours, even longer commutes, and more and more demands on precious family time are just a few of the variables that leave many of us feeling overwhelmed and exhausted at the end of the day.

In small doses, stress can actually be good for us. Stress gets the blood pumping and improves attention and concentration when it is experienced in small doses. At the other extreme, chronically high levels of stress can impair immune function, mood and wellbeing as individuals feel overwhelmed and out of control in their daily lives.

Different people respond differently to stress. Some become withdrawn and anxious, while others compensate with alcohol, drugs and food. For those who use food for comfort, the link between eating and stress is likely to have been formed when we were young. Crying babies are often soothed with food, when they may in fact be looking for touch and attention.

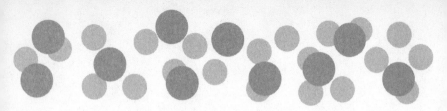

The issue with using food to help temporarily relieve stress is that we can, in turn, start to use stress as an excuse to eat poor quality food. If each and every time you feel a little frazzled you are stuffing a couple of chocolate biscuits into your mouth, this can quickly translate long-term into a couple of extra packets of biscuits a week. If such behaviours actually fixed the stress, perhaps there would be no issue, but in many cases, eating poor quality, high calorie food is likely to make your stress and anxiety worse.

If you are going through a stressful period it is worth considering the way you may use food to relieve your stress. More importantly, think about what nutrient-dense food choices you may need in your diet to help support your body during particularly stressful periods. Ideally, eating regularly with a balance of good quality carbohydrates and lean proteins will help to regulate your blood glucose levels and ensure you are at your best physically and mentally to deal with stress when it presents. Another simple trick is to be mindful of your use of stimulants such as coffee and cola-based drinks. While they may give you a hit of energy, they are also likely to give you a nasty energy lull an hour or so after consuming them, which may leave you less able to deal optimally with your stress. Aim for no more than two to three coffees a day and drink plenty of water to keep hydrated.

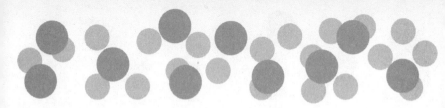

Stress places enormous demands on a number of the body's systems. Ensure your intake of key vitamins and minerals is optimal in order to proactively manage the stress in your life. In particular, the B group vitamins found in wholegrain breads and cereals are crucial for ensuring optimal energy, while the minerals iron and zinc will give your body the key nutrients it needs to produce red blood cells. If you are feeling chronically tired, and you know you don't eat as well as you should, taking a multivitamin can ensure you have an adequate intake of these key nutrients. If the fatigue is continual, it may also be worth taking a trip to your GP for a routine blood test to ensure everything is alright medically.

The most important thing to remember when it comes to stress and eating is that while the instant reward from consuming sweet foods can make us feel momentarily better, food is unable to solve the underlying issues that are causing stress or emotional distress. The key to ultimately managing stress-based eating is learning to adequately manage the stress itself. For many of us this means learning to cope better and develop clear strategies for identifying, managing and reducing the amount of stress in our daily lives.

Top 10 stress-less techniques

1 Move your body each day.
2 Express gratitude for something that is great in your life.
3 Take time out to chat to someone close to you each day.
4 Grow something.
5 Cut your TV viewing time by half.
6 Smile at one new person each day.
7 Phone a close friend.
8 Have a good belly laugh.
9 Do one nice thing for yourself each day.
10 Do something nice for someone else.

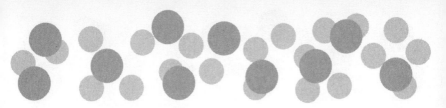

Travel smart

'Never let yourself become a victim of your environment.'

When busy professionals come in for an appointment, it is rarely a lack of knowledge preventing them from reaching their health and fitness goals. Rather it is a busy lifestyle and not paying enough attention to planning that sees them becoming a victim of their environment.

If you consider that the standard snack served on domestic flights contains more than 350 calories, or a quarter of a female's daily calorie requirement, and up to 60g of carbohydrate, or the equivalent of 4 slices of bread, it is easy to see where things can go off track so easily.

The way you can ensure that you keep on track with your diet and exercise regime, even if you travel regularly, is by keeping your food routine as stable as possible no matter where you're going. Always travel with protein-rich snacks and fruit, and get into the habit of saying no when other food is served, knowing it is unlikely to be of the quality you require. Make a concerted effort to get out of the hotel to a local supermarket to keep your breakfast foods and snacks on hand, and remember that if you're paying for hotel service, staff will often be more than happy to prepare the specific salads, wraps and even snacks you request, even if you have to pay a little extra for them.

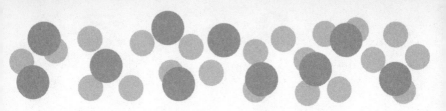

When it comes to work lunches, if they are pre-orders, put in a special dietary request in advance to ensure you will be served enough protein and salad or grab a sandwich or sushi in the morning to take with you. Eating out is no excuse. No matter which restaurant or food outlet you go to, there will be good choices. Base your meals around lean proteins and always order extra sides of vegetables or salad. You don't have to be a food purist if you're dining at a top restaurant as a one-off, but if you travel regularly you'll need to keep your dietary regime on track if you really want to lose or even just control your weight.

Another thing to remember is that for many of us, travelling actually provides an opportunity to move more. All of a sudden typical time drainers – including commuting, children and partners, or no easy access to a gym – are eliminated, making it far easier to find 30 minutes to get to the hotel gym or go for a quick walk before breakfast. Look to your travel time as an opportunity to move more, not less.

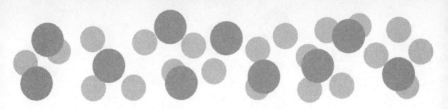

Get a daily timetable

'No time is a poor excuse – we all have 24 hours in a day. How do you use yours?'

Every single person I know is busy. How many people do you know who regularly say, 'I have a spare hour, what can I do with it?' Long working hours, long commutes, bulging social diaries all contribute to extremely full schedules and a constant lack of time to do the things that we really want to. In saying that, we all have 24 hours a day. Some of us manage to do a lot with that time and others far less, which means we need to be better with our time management if we are to fit regular exercise and healthy eating into our day.

An easy way to work out how you could become more efficient and free up some time for a healthy lifestyle is to work out where you currently spend your time and more importantly, where you waste it. Simply make a template of your entire 24 hours, and fill in the spaces over a week. The most common areas people waste time are watching mindless TV and the advertisements that go with it, commuting, getting out of bed late and surfing the internet. While there is nothing wrong with watching a little TV or relaxing, doing it out of habit and fatigue as opposed to interest is where we waste time.

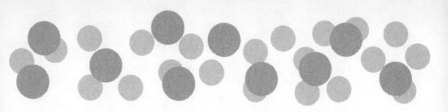

Once you are aware of where your time goes, you can start to develop strategies to become more efficient. Taping shows you like and watching them without the advertisements, trying to drive outside peak hour, getting up early and fitting in some exercise – all of these are examples of ways that busy people get things done in their world.

To really be in control of your weight and your body, you need to have a very clear idea of what you need to do each day to support your health goals, and how you are going to fit these things into your schedule. Once you are aware of these steps, documenting them and practising them until they become a daily habit will be the act that converts your health desires into your health outcomes.

So this week, as you sit at your computer with your morning coffee, start to make a list of all the things you need to do each day to make sure you eat well and exercise. Then factor all the items into your weekly timetable. Print it out and stick it up by your computer. A regular glance at it will remind you that you need to make yourself a cup of green tea, or walk upstairs to the bathroom to get your step number up. Remember, it's the little things that add up and lead to positive long-term health outcomes.

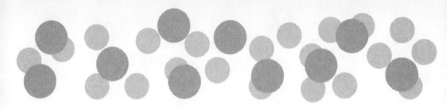

Sacred Sunday

*'Sunday is the day to get ready for the week ahead
so that come Monday you hit the ground running.'*

Sundays are often just as busy as every other day of the week with social functions and even work taking over this traditional day of rest. This usually means we fall into bed late on Sunday night, even more exhausted than we were on Friday, dreading the week ahead. If this sounds familiar, it's time to instate Sacred Sunday.

Sacred Sunday means setting aside one day every week when nothing is planned, so you can prepare for a healthy week ahead. You need to greet each Monday with a week's supply of healthy food so you start the week on the right foot. Sacred Sunday gives you time to shop for the food you need to eat well, time to prepare a couple of meals so you have some back-up options for those late nights home, and time to move your body. A good night's sleep on Sunday also makes you less likely to skip the all-important Monday workout.

Part of Sacred Sunday is also to set goals for the week, so as you relax in bed or in front of the TV, make a note of three to five things you hope to achieve in the week ahead. Small but steady and regular progress on our goals brings us closer to achieving them.

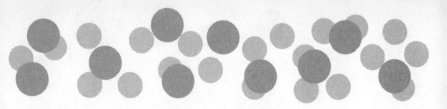

You have the power to manage your weight

'You now have the tools you need to manage your weight – the question is, will you choose to use them?'

As we approach the end of this book, you will have some new diet and lifestyle tricks that you've started to implement and that you will be able to maintain for many years to come. I also hope you come away feeling motivated and positive as you finally move forward with your health goals.

Although some of these new weight-loss tricks are exciting, deep down we all know how to look after our bodies. We know that we need to eat less and move more. We know that we need to cut back at times, and when we need to take our training or food choices to a new level. If we are truly honest with ourselves, we know what holds us back.

As is the case with any behavioural change process, you will make the changes at the exact time that things are right for you to do so. Listening and trusting yourself is often the step we need to take to cement things. So from today, know that you now have the knowledge, the tools and the mental strength you need to manage your weight. Once you cement this belief, you can only move forward.

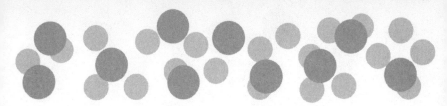

Victim no more

'I can never lose weight, it's not fair.'

The sooner you stop playing the weight-loss victim, the sooner you'll gain control of your weight, health and fitness. The same can be said for life – some of us are always the victim. We don't have enough money, time, hate our job, have an awful boyfriend holding us back, and the list goes on.

So, are you a victim of your own life? Do you constantly complain but do nothing to change your circumstance? Do you spend time with people who never tend to move forward? Do you bring energy to others or do you drain it?

Many of us earn a victim mentality when small via parents or early school experiences, but it's never too late to identify and make positive changes to reverse it.

When I first meet a new client in a weight-loss consultation, I can tell almost immediately if they are going to succeed with their weight loss goals. Individuals who are ready to change have a very different attitude to those who are there hoping that I will pull out my magical weight-loss wand and hit them on the head with it. Those who succeed are looking for the opportunity to get their weight under control, are open to new ideas and draw on their personal resources to be able to make the often simple life changes they need to take control.

The truth be known, we are all incredibly lucky – lucky to have the bodies we complain about, lucky to have easy access to good-quality food, lucky to have all the opportunities we easily take for granted. It's time to embrace that luck and think about ways we can make the most of it. To be grateful for the body we've been given, nurture it with good food and keep it healthy with plenty of movement. To accept that life in general is challenging but rewarding if we actively seek to improve it rather than wallow and complain.

There is no easy way out when it comes to weight control. The majority of us need to eat well most of the time and move regularly. It's as simple or complex as you choose to make it.

CHANGE YOUR MINDSET	
VICTIM RESPONSE	**OPPORTUNIST RESPONSE**
I wish I could eat what I want.	Few people can really eat what they want.
I can never lose weight.	Everyone can lose weight if they do it the right way for them.
I gain weight no matter what I eat.	You will only gain weight if you are eating too many calories.
Weight loss is so hard.	Everything is hard when you first start.
Weight loss should be easy.	The benefits of weight loss are too huge to miss out on.

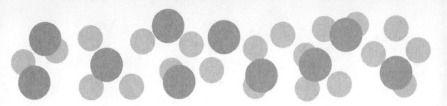

No more excuses

'Excuses – some of us make them, others take responsibility and refuse to bow down to them.'

Have you ever wondered why some people reach their goals and stay on track no matter what, and others always have an excuse why they haven't done what they said they would do? If you are really committed to getting your weight under control for good, you have to get rid of your excuses. No more excuses as to why you missed your workout. No more excuses as to why you ate rubbish for lunch. Why you skipped your walk. Why you did not have the foods at work you need to eat well.

Successful people do not make excuses. They do what they need to do to make sure things happen. They take charge and schedule training sessions they know they will get to. They prepare their food no matter where they are in the world. They work as hard as they need to get things done. And if and when they do occasionally go off track, they get right back on it.

Are you an excuse maker? Do you regularly change your schedule so that eating well and exercising take a back seat? Do you eat rubbish when you could have eaten better with a little extra effort and focus? One of the most common reasons we make excuses for not doing what we said we would is that the goals we have set are not in line with our own values and

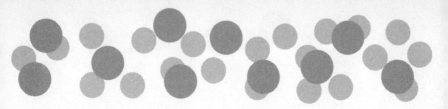

personal likes. We commit to a gym membership even though we hate the gym or try to follow a diet that we loathe. It's crucial to develop an eating plan and exercise regime that's realistic and right for you.

The next thing you can do to move away from the excuse mindset is to be aware of the times you are making excuses. When you feel an excuse coming on, rather than take the easy option, look for other alternatives to ensure you keep your lifestyle goals on track.

Once you eliminate the option for excuses, all of a sudden you are free from psychological limitations and can move forward with your weight loss. Remember that many of our behaviours are habits – habits that have become deeply entrenched after years of practice. If you have always come up with excuses that prevent you from reaching your weight-loss goals, they will keep popping up until you eradicate them. Don't give yourself a choice – just commit.

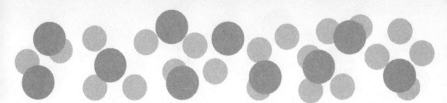

THE MOST COMMON EXCUSES

Not enough time 'There was no time', 'I ran out of time', or 'I just don't have time'. Hmm, who does? The funny thing about time is that we are all given the exact same amount of it. Ultimately it comes down to how we choose to spend our time. Maintaining a healthy lifestyle takes time – you need time to prepare and shop for food; you need time to exercise; and you need time to attend appointments that will help you to reach your goals. So if your excuse is that you do not have time to prepare food or get to the gym, it is simply not that big a priority at that time in your life. Individuals who maintain their weight, exercise regularly and eat well make time to do so.

Too tired The irony with blaming fatigue as a reason for not eating well or exercising is that the less you move and the poorer your diet, the more fatigued you are going to feel. Naturally, if you are feeling abnormally tired it is important that you make sure everything is fine medically, but if you are tired because you stay up too late, eat crappy food and sit down much more than you move, it is time to stop playing the victim. Make a commitment to get more sleep, eat a healthy diet and spend at least 20–30 minutes walking each day. These are all easy ways to help relieve fatigue the natural way.

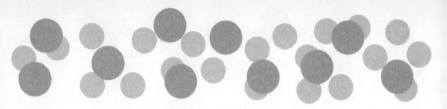

I'll start tomorrow Positive lifestyle changes do not occur with grandiose plans and unsustainable programs, rather they begin with you making each food and lifestyle decision a proactive, positive one. When clients bring in their food diaries with reports of fast-food and binge eating, the question needs to be asked, 'Why did you make that decision at that time?' Positive lifestyle change does not mean you have to be perfect. Rather it is about making strong food and exercise decisions more often than not.

It's too hard There is a common perception that some people have it easy when it comes to weight control. Clients constantly report that it is too hard to follow a program, or not fair that they have to be so strict. I would argue, however, that the majority of people who control their weight work pretty hard at it. Rather than focus on 'how hard' it is, instead focus on the benefits of looking after their body and how good it makes them feel. Eating well and exercising is as hard as you make it. The more you focus on how hard it is, the harder it will appear. Instead, focus on the positives of making healthy lifestyle changes and move forward.

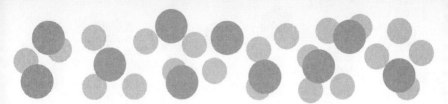

There is too much going on This is another good one: 'I went off track this week as there were too many things on.' Events, parties, celebrations, work drinks. Guess what? Chances are there will always be these types of events on, which means you will need to learn to manage yourself at them. Accept that going to an event or celebration does not mean you have to throw all diet structure out the window and binge eat. Nor does a busy diary mean you have to skip exercise altogether. Rather, it is about learning to control yourself and maintain a healthy diet platform and exercise regime, no matter how busy your diary is. Once you focus on what you need to do to achieve this balance, then the food and event distractions become less of a focus (and no longer act as a major excuse).

Rejecting laziness

'Are you tired? Overworked? Or are you just lazy?'

It's easy to be lazy living in a society where food is abundant and living standards are high. We leave garages and drive to offices with undercover parking. We have people to deliver our shopping, calculate our tax and take care of our dry cleaning, but when health or fitness professionals suggest moving our bodies more, we take the advice begrudgingly.

Living in a blessed world is sadly a large part of the reason so many of us are fat and unfit. We're quick to make excuses for not preparing our own food or to explain why we missed a gym session. We are quick to blame our laziness on fatigue or a low mood but the truth is to make long-term lifestyle changes that support weight control, we need to be strict, identify our lazy behaviour and put a stop to it.

Do you routinely switch off the morning alarm or cancel training sessions? Do you often find yourself eating fast food because you're too lazy to spend an extra 10 minutes preparing a more nutritious dinner? Do you grab quick high-fat snacks on the run because you are too lazy to go to the supermarket and stock up on more nutritious snack food options? We are all time poor and have a lot going on but some people manage to get things done and keep their diet on track, and some don't. Which do you want to be?

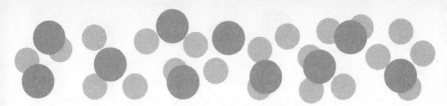

See only solutions

*'I don't want to hear what went badly,
I only want to hear what went well.'*

When clients return for a weight loss review after their first appointment,
it's common for them to spend the first few minutes outlining all the
things they've done wrong or not completed. The scary thing is that
starting any dialogue with such a negative mindset has been proven to
narrow our brain's ability to identify opportunities and strategies to move
forward. We talk ourselves into failure.

It is imperative when committing to long-term behavioural change and
sustainable weight loss that we remain solution-focused at all times – that
is, looking only for answers, not problems. Seeking ways to move forward
rather than dwelling on what has not come together, seeking answers to
apparent problems rather than complaining, being on the constant look
out for new opportunities, for good to come from apparent bad, being
positive, all the time.

It's very easy to fall into old thought patterns and habits when it comes to
weight loss; 'Weight loss is so hard', 'I can never lose weight', 'Diets never
work for me', or 'I don't have time for exercise'. Each of these declarations
is negative in both tone and direction. A simple shift towards the positive,
'This time I will lose weight for good', 'This time I will lose weight no

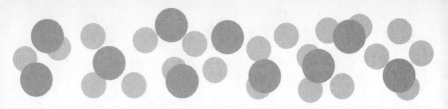

matter what', 'I will find the right dietary balance for me', 'I will find time to exercise every day', is all you need to start looking for opportunities to control your weight as opposed to reasons not to.

If you think about it, the role of a health professional in the weight loss process is simply to help brainstorm ideas that will help you progress. To think about dietary options and new foods to try that will help achieve the ideal dietary balance, to brainstorm new exercise options, to support, problem solve and move you forward. And you too can do this simply by always remaining solution-focused on your weight-loss journey. Waste no time dwelling on problems that arise – instead view them as a way to take the next step and move forward. Know that there is always an answer and that road humps are simply part of any change and new process.

Once you adopt a solution-only approach you will be surprised how much easier life becomes. Precious time and energy is no longer wasted on things we cannot control, but channelled into making our goals achieveable.

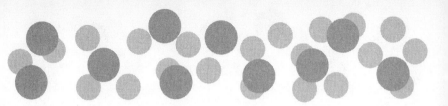

Commit to self-care

'Be your best for you, and then for those around you.'

Men are much better at it than women, and mothers are the worst of all. Our weight, mood and health suffer when we don't do it, but it can be a challenging habit to build and maintain – self-care. Although it seems like a basic biological function, much time is spent in diet consultations helping people learn the importance of self-care – the daily need to keep body, mood and health in good shape so we can be at our best.

The mistake many of us make is not prioritising our own needs, instead giving everything to others before we consider caring for ourselves. This leaves us tired, grumpy, overweight and resentful while teaching others that this is okay, so friends and family continue to expect it. If you know you need to work on your self-care, here are some starting ideas:

1 Aim for at least one fun social event each week.
2 Aim to do one nice thing for yourself each week.
3 Aim for some alone time with your partner at least once a month.
4 Schedule at least three exercise sessions each week.
5 Plan at least one break or holiday to look forward to each year.

Once you create these breaks in your life, you'll be surprised how much better you feel, and how much more energy you have to make the effort to eat well and move your body.

Commit to a steely mindset

'Allow nothing to distract you from your health and lifestyle goals.'

Life is full of distractions – situations, people and opportunities that cross our path on an hourly, daily, yearly basis. We can either choose to engage with them or continue along our self-directed path. Some people are exceptionally good at ignoring distractions, quickly determining whether they are in line with their big picture plan. Others spend their lives being distracted by other people or life in general and never really achieve any of their goals. These people often feel unsatisfied and unfulfilled, wondering where on earth the time went, and why they're in exactly the same place they were 5 years ago.

The same can be said for those people who manage to stay on track with their weight-loss goals and those who don't. People who stay on track don't skip their walk or workout for a shopping trip. They say no to an extra glass of wine or dessert because they know what they need to do to stay healthy and feel good.

Developing a steely mindset when it comes to your food and training regimes will take time, especially if it's a new thing for you. First of all it will require you to clearly define your goals. Next you need to identify distracters – the people, events, media and other stimuli that take you off track, physically or mentally, and develop strategies to ignore them. Learn

to avoid and ignore the countless hours of mindless chatter with people who will not be a part of your life long-term, to avoid and ignore the constant media stream in which we waste so much time and energy, to avoid and ignore people in our world who drain our energy and leave us less inclined to go about achieving our goals.

At times this may mean missing social engagements we didn't want to go to anyway, or that we have no idea what's happening on the latest TV show, but it will also mean we have more time to look after ourselves. And the more we nurture and look after ourselves, the better the position we find ourselves in to manage our weight long-term.

Identifying distracters

- Will I have any regrets if I don't participate in this event?
- Will this person be in my life in 1, 5 or 10 years?
- What could I achieve if I don't do this?
- What is the most important thing I can do with my time right now?
- In my life, which people, events and activities bring me the most pleasure?
- What's the worst thing that can happen if I don't do this?

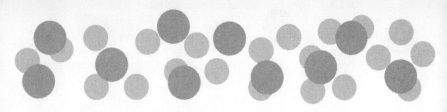

Cement your new habits

'It takes 3 days to become aware of a new habit and up to 3 months before an old habit is replaced, so be patient.'

Habits – the things we do day in, day out without thinking – are crucial when it comes to developing sustainable diet and exercise changes. Developing a new habit is all very well but cementing it to become a long-term regular part of your day is something else. Now you have come this far, here are the key habits that we know are linked to weight control long-term and that you need to cement if you are to improve your food, your body and your life, for good.

1. ALWAYS EAT BREAKFAST

People who eat a substantial breakfast lose more weight than those who have a small breakfast. Choose eggs or baked beans on wholegrain bread, natural muesli with fruit and yoghurt or a liquid meal drink and notice how much more satisfied you feel throughout the morning.

2. EAT 3 CUPS OF VEGETABLES AND TWO FRUITS EACH DAY

Having half your plate filled with vegetables or salad at lunch and dinner helps to tick this box, as does adding fruit to your breakfast and vegetable for a snack on the way home from work.

3. TAKE TIME TO SHOP EACH WEEK

If the food is not in the house, how can you eat well? Schedule in time to shop each week and use online options if you hate spending time in a busy supermarket.

4. WALK 10,000 STEPS A DAY

Remember this is on top of your regular exercise routine. A pedometer is extremely useful in providing feedback on how many steps you are racking up every day.

5. SIT DOWN AT THE TABLE TO EAT

You will eat more slowly and often eat less food as a result. Remember eating is supposed to be an enjoyable and social experience so take time out to do it properly.

6. ALWAYS CARRY A HEALTHY SNACK

Most of us know what the good food choices are – the problem arises when we get hungry and don't have nutritious food options with us and end up eating high-fat food on the run. Great options to keep handy include nut or protein snack bars, hard fruit (such as an apple) or a few crackers so you're never caught off guard.

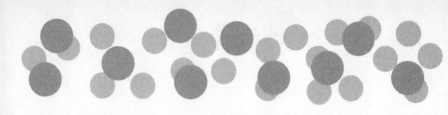

7. DRINK GREEN TEA AFTER MEALS

Not only is green tea exceptionally high in antioxidants, it can also help increase metabolic rate and curb sugar cravings.

8. ALWAYS CARRY A WATER BOTTLE

Once again, if it's in front of you, you will drink it. Aim for at least two bottles of water each day as a replacement for juice, cordial or soft drink.

9. CHOOSE WHOLEGRAIN, LOW-GI BREAD AND CEREALS

Aim for the best quality bread, crackers and breakfast cereal as these are foods we eat every day. Choose low-GI, wholegrain pastas, cereals and breads that are portion-controlled such as small slices of grain bread and measured serves of breakfast cereal, rice and pasta.

10. EAT CARBS AND PROTEIN FOR OPTIMAL SATIETY

Low-GI carbohydrates provide sustainable energy, while protein offers key nutrients and helps to keep us full. Some examples are eggs on grain toast, yoghurt and fruit, crackers and cheese or wholegrain bread with tuna, chicken or salmon.

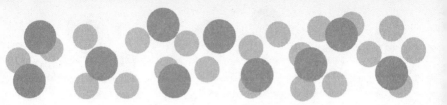

Maintain your motivation

'You can have anything if you want it enough.'

Motivation is a complex and changeable state. For many, it's innate when it comes to health and fitness. For others, a health scare or realisation that they're four sizes bigger than they should be provides the kick needed to turn their lives around. Then there are those who just never get it. They try one health and fitness craze after the other, never cementing a pattern of living that works for them and gives their bodies a better chance.

If you have reached this point in the book, it's safe to say that you're motivated and keen to stay that way. To achieve your goals, you'll need strategies to maintain this motivation by regularly reminding yourself why you've committed to important diet and exercise changes long-term. Some simple questions that may help you to clarify your reasons for wanting to stay fit and healthy include:

- What are the benefits of keeping my body fit and healthy?
- How would my life be better if I felt better about my body?
- Am I a healthy role model for my children?
- Can I physically do all the things I would like to?
- If I was fit, healthy and happy what would I be eating and what training would I be doing each day?
- If I knew I could help keep my body disease-free by eating well and exercising, would I be more inclined to move more and eat less?

- Who are the people in my life who would support me living like this?
- What changes can I make to my lifestyle today that will help move me closer to my goal of living well and feeling good?

Having clear answers to these questions reminds you of the bigger reasons for wanting to get in shape and stay there. Keep these answers on hand and refer back to them if you find yourself going off track. A simple and proven technique to maintain motivation for healthy living is to make a visual reminder of these questions and answers and place them somewhere where you will see them every day. When we repeatedly remind ourselves of the reasons why we make simple daily decisions, it helps reinforce the key behaviours and habits we need to stay on track. Keep a copy of these mantras at work, in the car and on your mobile phone so you can take control and pull yourself back in line.

For behavioural change to be sustained long-term, the reason for wanting it in the first place needs to come from within. It cannot be based on wanting to look good for a wedding or to fit into a certain dress – the motivation has to become so entrenched that you can no longer imagine life without it. As you embrace this new approach to weight loss and start to take control of your health, give yourself 3 months to cement your new habits. Then the longer you maintain these habits after that 3-month period, the harder they will be to break.

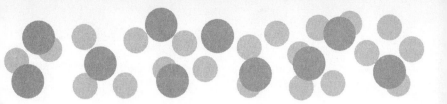

Embrace your true self

'Be kind to yourself.'

Time after time, seasoned dieters attend a new diet appointment or read another magazine and mentally commit to the latest diet or training program. Yet after a day, week or month, the regime falls apart and they're back to where they started, feeling worse about themselves than ever before. It's an exhausting, boring, predictable cycle that achieves nothing.

The most important step you can take towards ending this vicious cycle is to be kind to yourself. Consider what you really need – from your relationships, work, social life and diet and exercise regime. Figuring this out has to come from approaching self-care positively, not from a position of frustration where you beat yourself up for being fat and lazy. The negative mindset instantly talks you into failure and gives you excuses to revert to old habits. So don't punish yourself – give yourself a break.

Once you start being kind to yourself and nourishing your mind and body with exercise and the right amount of good-quality food, you'll be in the perfect position to determine the best way forward in looking after yourself for life. You will move beyond the diet and exercise baggage that has literally weighed you down for too long and enjoy the lifestyle that makes you feel good. You are free to enjoy what life has waiting for you – so get on with it, the time is now.

This edition published in 2018 by Hardie Grant Books,
an imprint of Hardie Grant Publishing

First published in 2011

Hardie Grant Books (Melbourne)
Building 1, 658 Church Street
Richmond, Victoria 3121

Hardie Grant Books (London)
5th and 6th Floors
52–54 Southwark Street
London SE1 1UN

www.hardiegrant.com

A Cataloguing-in-Publication data is available from the National Library of
Australia at www.nla.gov.au

Losing the Last 5 kg: Simple steps to get the body you want now
ISBN 9781743794289

Cover design by Kate Barraclough
Text design and typesetting by Jacqueline Richards and Megan Ellis
Printed by McPherson's Printing Group, Maryborough, Victoria